The Search for Health Needs

Also by Sarah Cowley:

Norman, I. and Cowley, S. (1999) *The Changing Nature of Nursing in a Managerial Age.* Blackwell Science, Oxford

The Search for Health Needs

Research for health visiting practice

Edited by

Jane V. Appleton and Sarah Cowley

6,7,12,77, 85

First published 2000 by
MACMILLAN PRESS LTD
Houndmills, Basingstoke, Hampshire RG21 6XS
and London
Companies and representatives throughout the world

ISBN 0–333–72144–6

A catalogue record for this book is available from the British Library.

This book is printed on paper suitable for recycling and made from fully managed and sustained forest sources.

10   9   8   7   6   5   4   3   2   1
09   08   07   06   05   04   03   02   01   00

Editing and origination by
Aardvark Editorial, Mendham, Suffolk

Printed in Malaysia

Contents

List of contributors

Jane V. Appleton is Principal Lecturer in Nursing at the University of Hertfordshire.

Jenny Billings is Lecturer in the Research in Nursing Studies Section at King's College London.

Clare Blackburn is Senior Research Fellow in the Department of Social Studies at the University of Warwick.

Sarah Cowley is Professor of Community Practice Development at King's College London.

Amanda Kelsey is Lecturer in Community Nursing at the University of York.

Ina Machen is Senior Lecturer in Nursing at the University of Hertfordshire.

Sheila Twinn is Senior Lecturer in Nursing at the Chinese University of Hong Kong.

Preface

The contentious nature of the term 'health needs' surfaced along with the debates about prioritising and rationing the NHS that followed the introduction of the NHS and Community Care Act 1990. Under the legislation, 'health needs' were distinguished and separated from 'social needs' (DoH 1989a, 1989b). In the NHS, purchasing authorities were established that were, with guidance from their medical Directors of Public Health, responsible for assessing the health needs of the local population and purchasing services to meet those needs from separate provider units. At an individual level, care managers were to assess the needs and circumstances of people with disabilities, the elderly and the mentally ill, and then purchase suitable 'packages of care' as indicated by their assessments. Distinguishing between health and social needs was paramount as that distinction determined whether the responsibility for meeting the cost of service provision should fall to the NHS or the local authority social services.

Given the importance of this distinction, it is perhaps a little surprising that the legislation provided no definition of the terms 'health need' and 'social need'; it does, however, go some way towards explaining why the term 'need' became the focus of much discussion and debate. As this text goes to press, new legislation (the Health Bill 1999) is progressing through parliament. This will retain the division between purchasing (to be known in future as 'commissioning') and providing authorities in the NHS (DoH, 1997). The emphasis on the provision of services to meet assessed needs will remain, and there is a commitment to breaking down the barriers between health and social care. There is still, however, no formal definition of what counts as an official 'need' for which a service must be provided.

The interest of health visitors in the notion of health needs has long preceded this recent legislative focus, and these professionals have traditionally viewed the term far more widely than as purely a mechanism for determining rights and responsibilities in relation to service provision. Health visiting developed as part of the public health movement in the middle of the nineteenth century. Although the occupation has become increasingly intertwined with nursing as the twentieth century has progressed, its practice has mirrored changes in the wider public health sphere (Cowley, 1996), and health visitors have throughout their history maintained a distinct, primary focus on prevention and health promotion. The Council for the Education and Training of Health Visitors (CETHV), which served as the regulating body for the profession from 1962 to 1983, provided a definition of the service that explains how this preventive emphasis necessarily includes a broad understanding of health and health needs. They indicated that (CETHV, 1977: 8):

> The professional practice of health visiting consists of planned activities aimed at the promotion of health and prevention of ill health. It therefore contributes substantially to individual and social well-being, by focusing attention at various times on either an individual, a social group or a community. It has three unique functions:
>
> Identifying and fulfilling self-declared as well as unrecognised health needs of individuals and social groups.
>
> Providing a generalist health agent service in an era of increasing specialisation in the health care available to individuals and communities.
>
> Monitoring simultaneously the health needs and demands of individuals and communities; contributing to the fulfilment of these needs; and facilitating appropriate care and services by other professional health care groups.

The service was to be delivered by implementing certain principles in practice, the first of which was the 'search for health needs' (CETHV, 1977). This volume has brought together a collection of research that helps to explain both the breadth of meaning in this phrase and its continuing contemporary relevance. The first chapter provides more information about the principles of health visiting, setting them in the context of current public health and primary health care practice. Although the principles were originally devised for use by one occupational group, this collection of research demonstrates their wider utility and potential for use across agencies and disciplines as public health and health promotion are emphasised in the new legislative agenda. Furthermore, by illustrating a range of research approaches to investigate the 'search for health needs', it is hoped that this volume will stimulate debate and further research as well as providing a basis to guide and inform community nursing and health visiting practice.

SARAH COWLEY AND JANE V. APPLETON

References

Council for the Education and Training of Health Visitors (CETHV) (1977) *An Investigation into the Principles of Health Visiting.* London: CETHV (reprinted 1993, English National Board for Nursing, Midwifery and Health Visiting, London).

Cowley S. (1996) Reflecting on the past; preparing for the next century. *Health Visitor* **69**(8): 313–16.

Department of Health (DoH) (1989a) *Working for Patients.* Cmnd 555. London: HMSO.

Department of Health (DoH) (1989b) *Caring for People.* Cmnd 849. London: HMSO.

Department of Health (DoH) (1997) *The New NHS: Modern, Dependable.* Cmnd 3809. London: Stationery Office.

Acknowledgements

The authors and publishers wish to thank the following for permission to use copyright material:

Macmillan Press for material based on Appleton J.V. (1997) Establishing the validity and reliability of clinical practice guidelines used to identify families requiring increased health visitor support. *Public Health* **111**:107–13.

Blackwell Science for material based on Appleton J.V. and Cowley S. (1997) Analysing clinical practice guidelines. A method of documentary analysis. *Journal of Advanced Nursing* **25**: 1008–17 and Machen I. (1996) The relevance of health visiting policy to contemporary mothers. *Journal of Advanced Nursing* **24**: 350–6.

English National Board for Nursing, Midwifery and Health Visiting for Figure 1.1 from Bergen *et al.* (1996) An investigation into the changing educational needs of community nurses with regards to needs assessment and quality care in the context of the NHS and Community Care Act 1990.

Every effort has been made to contact all copyright holders but if any have been inadvertently omitted the publishers will be pleased to make the necessary arrangement at the earliest opportunity.

1

The Search for Health Needs

Sarah Cowley and Jane V. Appleton

The widely recognised assumption that health is the absence of disease has underpinned successive health service policies; this medical model approach is significant for a number of professional groups involved in health promotion and for the population itself. In particular, it is relevant to service definitions and functions carried out by health visitors, whose practice has adopted a more holistic approach and consists of planned activities aimed at the promotion of health and the prevention of ill health (CETHV, 1977). At present, all children under school age and their families are allocated to a health visiting caseload for purposes of health promotion and preventive care; other age groups may be included depending on local policies.

However, if need is construed as the presence of a disease or (at least) as a problem that is amenable to change by health service intervention, only individuals with specified illnesses or risks are viewed as a legitimate focus for attention in a 'needs-led' health service. In such formulations, the well population is perceived as having no potential to benefit from health promotion or the attention of health professionals. Such reasoning has been used to justify a dramatic reduction in health visiting services directed at the well population. It is assumed that families who display no overt problems at a single encounter (a first visit, used to 'assess needs') have no need for a health-promoting service and therefore should not be visited on a regular or routine basis (NHSE, 1996). This purchasing guidance contradicts the emerging public health agenda, which takes a far broader stance (DoH, 1998), yet it draws attention to the contested nature of health need and health service provision.

This volume offers a collection of different pieces of research that are all related to 'the search for health needs' (CETHV, 1977). This introductory chapter will begin by analysing the relevance of health needs in the current policy agenda, with particular reference to health visiting and public health. The longstanding interest of health visitors in this topic will be outlined before going on to explain how the 'search for health needs' was identified as a principle of health visiting. This principle holds a surface resonance with contemporary intentions to assess needs prior to planning or delivering services to meet them, but, as this volume will demonstrate, the search for health needs is not limited to a single step in the cycle of service planning.

Health needs

Health visiting has it roots firmly based in public health, having developed within the philanthropic sanitary reform movements in the middle of the nineteenth century. History shows that public health has moved from a radical, reforming focus on structural and environmental change in the middle of the nineteenth century, towards personal preventive activities, before emphasising therapeutic interventions by the mid-twentieth century (Ashton and Seymour, 1988).

Cowley (1996) suggests that health visiting has mirrored these changes over time. The practical, radical outlook with which the occupation began (Dingwall, 1977) gave way to the stereotype of 'the mother and baby nurse' when public health took on an increasingly individualistic focus between the two World Wars. By the 1970s, the profession began to question and articulate the basis of its work, identifying health and health needs as significant, if complex, underlying concepts (CETHV, 1977). At this time, the narrow, disease-focused approach to public health was being increasingly criticised for avoiding wider social issues and influences on health that lay beyond health service provision (Ashton and Seymour, 1988).

Even so, it was not until 1998 that a UK government finally acknowledged the importance to public health of wider influences such as poverty, homelessness and unemployment (DoH, 1998). These proposals stress the preventive importance of identifying and changing the root causes of ill health, although there is no new definition of how 'health needs' are to be regarded. Despite the fact that it was not defined, the concept of health need underpinned the NHS and Community Care Act 1990, which highlighted the importance of effectively assessing needs prior to planning and delivering services to meet them (DoH, 1989). This legislation created health authorities that were to assess the health needs of the population they served and then purchase services relevant to these identified needs. It distinguished firmly between 'health and social need' but did not clarify how these distinctions should be made.

The Health Bill 1999, currently before parliament, proposes to dismantle this internal market and promote collaboration between the health and social services. Separate health and social service budgets will remain, as will the divisions between the commissioners and providers of services (DoH, 1997). There is a new, formal role for community nurses in Primary Care Groups (PCGs), whose commissioning function may be seen as an extension of general practitioner (GP) fundholding. It is intended that these local organisations will contribute to the wider health improvement programmes developed by health authorities; the assumption is that GPs and community nurses are well placed to know about the health needs in their immediate area. Once more, the policy fails to specify what counts as a 'need' or how it should be defined, but the amount of debate triggered by the NHS and Community Care Act 1990 has contributed to a wider understanding of the concept.

One much-cited definition capturing the spirit of that earlier legislation suggested that need is 'the ability to benefit from health care' (Stevens and Gabbay, 1991: 20). Similarly, Rees-Jones (1995) viewed 'needs' only as 'health care needs', assessments being embedded in contracts for health services and service specifications. Both definitions link need firmly to health service provision and resource allocation. Arguably, a wider view is needed to account for the expanding public health agenda being proposed in *Our Healthier Nation* (DoH, 1998).

Health needs assessment can be defined as 'identifying an achievable change or changes which will improve health or health care' (Summers and McKeown, 1996: 323). This definition provides a starting point for identifying health outcomes. Measuring changes that occur as a result of clinical interventions for people with specific needs makes it possible to accrue evidence that the health care offered is effective in creating a beneficial change in health status. However, there is a dearth of information about how health needs should be specified in relation to health promotion within the well population, in whom no actual change in individual health status is sought even if a general health benefit might somehow accrue. A different way of accounting for both health needs and outcomes is required for this public health approach.

Thus, confusion surrounds the term 'need', and the literature continues to describe it as a contested concept (Buchan *et al.*, 1990; Stevens and Gabbay, 1991; Billings and Cowley, 1995). Orr (1992: 115) has stated that need:

> is social in being defined according to standards of communal life, relative in that its mean will vary from age to age and from society to society, and evaluative in that it is based on value judgements.

As this excerpt suggests, health visitors recognise that health and social need are often inextricably linked. However, a concept of health need that encompasses poverty and social issues contrasts with the narrow medical model approach that focuses solely on disease; this creates potential difficulties for a health visiting service that depends for funding upon a highly medicalised health service.

Carney *et al.* (1996) have suggested that health visitors identify needs at both the community level, in terms of health profiling, and the level of the individual; they argue that health visitors should develop skills in both areas. Bergen *et al.* (1996) have similarly examined and clarified the meaning of 'needs assessment' from an educational viewpoint. An analysis of their focus group data indicates that the term 'need' is perceived as a 'dual concept', one element reflecting its subjectivity and personal nature, the other that some aspects of need are more explicit and measurable. Despite the contradictory nature of these two elements, Bergen *et al.* (1996) argue that both are integral to the concept of need. In turn, needs assessment involves three aspects:

- the recognition of needs;
- the assessment of needs;
- linking the assessment of needs to the ongoing process of service planning.

Like Carney *et al.* (1996), Bergen *et al.* have suggested that these assessments apply at the level of individuals, families, caseload or local area and wider population groups. Summers and McKeown (1996) insist that health visitors must recognise that they have the skills and knowledge to provide sound evidence that their service is, and can be, responsive to local health and social needs; they are in an ideal position to identify, access and collate public health data sources, reflecting local needs. However, Bergen *et al.* (1996) found that practitioners were not encouraged to (and were sometimes actively discouraged from) developing profiles of health needs in the area in which they worked; this was frequently viewed as a managerial or purchasing function (Figure 1.1).

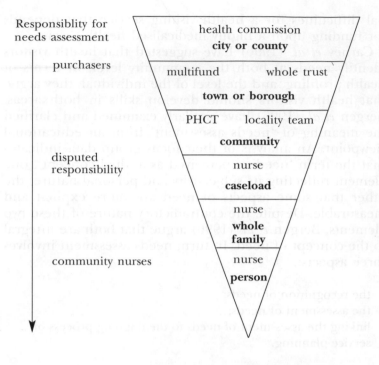

Responsiblity for needs assessment

purchasers

disputed responsibility

community nurses

health commission
city or county

multifund   whole trust
town or borough

PHCT   locality team
community

nurse
caseload

nurse
whole family

nurse
person

Figure 1.1   Responsibility for needs assessment
(from Bergen *et al.*, 1996)

Health visiting and health needs

This controversy about who takes responsibility for health needs assessment draws attention to the lack of legitimacy associated with much health visiting work and the importance of recognising the function of the role. It suggests that much of the debate surrounding ways of distinguishing health and social need, of 'proper' approaches to needs assessment and appropriate ways of recognising 'real needs', is a covert approach to rationing service provision. Many families depend on the services that health visitors and school nurses offer; this is particularly true of vulnerable groups – families with young children who are socially

isolated or living in poverty, women with depression and
those who are subjected to violence and intimidation
(Symonds, 1997). In reality, no other preventive services
are there to support these people (DoH, 1995; Appleton,
1996), so there is an urgent need to prove the value of
these community nursing services. Research can be a way
to demonstrate these 'real needs' (Symonds, 1997) and
assess the impact of nursing services on community life.

Indeed, if need is a contested concept, so too is the role
and function of health visiting. In its early years, the occupation was strongly associated with the work of sanitary
inspectors, who evolved into today's environmental health
officers (Davies, 1988). As it developed in the early years
of the twentieth century, health visiting was closely linked
with state intervention in preventive and public health
issues (Dingwall, 1982; Robinson, 1982; SNMAC, 1995).
Health visiting became intertwined with nursing and child
health between the two World Wars, Dingwall (1977) asso-
ciating this change with a loss of the radicalism that characterised the early years of the profession.

By 1962, nursing and midwifery qualifications were
formally required for entry to the profession. Health visitors were employed by local authorities at that time; this
requirement was perhaps a defensive move in the light of
the growing power and higher academic level of social
workers (Robinson, 1982). More recently, loss of identity
within the wider nursing profession has seemed a greater
threat, given the force of recommendations to eliminate
state registration and the status of health visiting as a separate profession (J.M. Consulting, 1998). The government
rejected this proposal (HSC, 1999), but other difficulties
remain. As a legacy of fundholding, health visitors are nearly
all attached to general practices, which has led to increasing
medicalisation of the service (Symonds, 1997). Health
visitor education has been seriously reduced in length and
scope, being confined within a general community nursing
framework (UKCC, 1994). Unless they are additionally
registered as nurses, midwives are not entitled to register
as health visitors, even if they successfully complete the
training (UKCC, 1998). These combined influences are

creating much concern and renewed pressure for a direct entry route for health visitor students once more (for example Mackereth, 1997; Rowbotham, 1998).

However, such uncertainties seem to have been the lot of health visitors throughout their history. In 1974, the health visiting service was transferred from local authority responsibility to the auspices of the NHS along with public health medicine and community nursing. As the NHS had previously been concerned only with hospital services, this move created much anxiety. Recognising the potential difficulties, the Council for the Education and Training of Health Visitors (CETHV), which at that time regulated health visiting, set up a series of working groups to investigate the principles that underpinned the work. This 'working group' approach to discovering and articulating a professional consensus on the necessary knowledge, principles and practice of health visiting became a recurring feature (Table 1.1).

Table 1.1   Identifying the principles for practice

Publication	Working Group
Investigation into the principles and practice of health visiting (CETHV, 1977)	Working group initially convened by CETHV in 1974, comprising mainly educationalists but also including management representation
The investigation debate (CETHV, 1980)	A collection of papers and responses from a series of conferences convened by CETHV, discussions and debates held around the country
Principles in practice (CETHV, 1982)	Papers from the continuing debate and a workshop convened by CETHV and attended by practitioners, teachers and managers
A re-examination of the principles of health visiting (Twinn and Cowley, 1992)	Working group comprising practitioners, teachers, managers and researchers jointly convened by UK Standing Conference on Health Visitor Education (UKSC) with Health Visitors' Association (HVA)
Weights and measures: outcomes and evaluation in health visiting (Campbell *et al.*, 1995)	Working group comprising practitioners, teachers, managers and researchers, convened by Health Visitors' Association (HVA)

Health visiting and the concept of health

The 'investigation' set in train by the CETHV (1977) identified health as an individual and community value and
talked about how that view linked with the work of health
visitors, underpinning the idea of 'health need' and health
promotion that was held to be central to the work. Despite
recurrent warnings that 'health' represents too nebulous
and uncertain a concept to underpin a profession (Clough,
1980; Robinson, 1985), it continued to be regarded as an
important basic value. A later working group outlined seven
important beliefs about health that reinforced this as a
fundamental value underpinning health visiting practice
(Twinn and Cowley, 1992: 6–7). In summary these are:

1. Everyone has a fundamental right to the best possible state
   of health. In accepting this, health visitors take on a responsibility to address current health inequalities and inequities in
   health care.
2. Health promotion is important because having a positive sense
   of health enables people to make full use of their physical,
   mental and emotional capacities so that they can reach their
   full potential for achievement.
3. Achieving health means that people have the power to shape
   their own lives and those of their families. This implies an
   active participation in health by individuals, families and
   groups, and emphasises the importance of empowering as a
   form of health promotion.
4. Health care services should be readily accessible and
   acceptable, and involve full community participation. This is
   the basis of primary health care, which needs a full, equal
   partnership between professionals and the people they serve.
5. Health is a positive concept, encompassing social and
   personal resources as well as physical capacities. Resources
   that contribute to positive well-being may be personal and
   internalised, or may arise externally from the social and
   family context in which the individual lives. Health
   promotion therefore involves finding ways to create resources
   for health.

6. Health cannot be separated from the socioeconomic and cultural context in which it is experienced. This is why health visitors focus at different times on individuals, families or communities.
7. Health must be regarded in broad, holistic terms, encompassing whole individuals within their personal situation. This has implications for the extent to which people are able to exercise personal choice and to which they can be held solely responsible for their state of health.

These beliefs suggest that the concept of health cannot be viewed in isolation as it is inextricably linked with many social, cultural, political and economic issues. Twinn and Cowley (1992) describe how these fundamental beliefs reflect humanitarian principles that may be at odds with the market-led view of health as a commodity. Indeed, Cowley (1997) suggests that each of the key points listed may lead to difficulties in implementing the principles in practice.

The principles of health visiting

The working group convened in 1974 considered that health as a value underpinned the practice of health visiting, which, they suggested, was carried out through four principles describing the process of the work (CETHV, 1977):

1. the search for health needs;
2. the stimulation of the awareness of health needs;
3. the influence on policies affecting health;
4. the facilitation of health-enhancing activities.

When they were re-examined by a later working group of practitioners, educationalists and managers, these principles were found to be as relevant as ever to the health visiting profession (Twinn and Cowley, 1992). The initial work was intended for use in curriculum development, to inform the education and training of health visiting students, but when the CETHV was disbanded in 1983, the momentum of the work was lost. At that time, the regulation of the profession became the responsibility of the United Kingdom Central Council for Nursing, Midwifery and Health Visiting (UKCC). This organisation initially adapted the principles in a general framework for community nursing education (UKCC, 1994). This general usage might have been viewed as a testimony to the robust and forward-looking nature of the work undertaken by the CETHV (1977): it was a move that undoubtedly helped to overcome resistance from health visitors to the major changes in their professional preparation. However, a subsequent review removed the adapted version of the principles as required learning outcomes (UKCC, 1998), perhaps revealing that their initial inclusion may have been based more on a desire to reduce and confine health visiting within a nursing framework than to develop the profession and share its slightly different knowledge base across the community practice sphere.

However, it should not be supposed that the principles remain static and unchanging. The idea of seeking consensus across the profession on the values and principles that underpin the work differs radically from the approach used to determine the knowledge base in the wider nursing profession. The working group convened in 1991 confirmed their continued relevance but also developed the profession's understanding of the principles. A broader view of how they could be implemented began, as did the process of drawing on research to develop their meaning (Twinn and Cowley, 1992). Given the extent of change since that time, another 're-examination' may be called for. Alternatively, the 'working group approach' might represent a formative stage of defining professional knowledge, one that is now giving way to a more sophisticated, research-based process.

Researching the principles

There has been very little empirical work that explicitly uses the principles of health visiting as a basis for research, but there is a growing body of qualitative data that sheds light on their interpretation in practice. Twinn (1991, 1993), for example, incorporated the principles as an underlying philosophy for the conceptual framework that emerged from her research on how health visiting is interpreted in practice. The principles are not discrete or sequential: they overlap in practice, and much of the research can be regarded as contributing to an understanding of more than one sphere of practice. Even so, it is possible to see a pattern of emerging research activity.

'Facilitation'

The idea of the 'facilitation of health-enhancing activities' encompasses a potentially vast range of interventions, many of which could be examined from the viewpoint of health promotion or health education. Pearson (1991), for example, drew on a series of case studies of health visitors working with the mothers of new babies, identifying 'development' as a central theme that underpinned the role. Importantly, this study showed how relationships between health visitors and their clients changed and developed over time. The development of the baby was another key theme, as was development of the mother, both as a mother and as a person in her own right. Various authors have extended this educational process to encompass whole communities as health visiting embraces community development as a legitimate strategy through which to facilitate health-enhancing activities (for example Boyd *et al.*, 1993; Craig 1996; Brown, 1997).

Behavioural difficulties are commonly encountered in childhood, and research has shown that health visitors can effectively facilitate good parenting skills (Angeli, 1994; Pritchard, 1994; Davis *et al.*, 1997; Kerr *et al.* 1997). Even so, there is some concern that (unless it is equitably and sensitively handled) such health education might be an inappropriate substitute for providing practical help and access to relief from structural disadvantage (Edwards and Popay, 1994; Edwards, 1995). Similarly, children living in unsafe and inadequate home environments are more vulnerable to accidents in childhood, and an increasing body of work is available on the effectiveness of home support and health visiting intervention in reducing their prevalence (for example Colver *et al.*, 1982; Crew and Fletcher, 1995; Roberts *et al.*, 1996). Again, community-based interventions are beginning to emerge as preferable as they are less stigmatising than individual interventions and likely to be more effective in the long term (Coombes, 1991; Roberts *et al.*, 1993). Government proposals to introduce a specified range of such services for infants under the age of 4 years and their families within 'Surestart' centres that target small, local areas are intended to combine the non-stigmatising benefit of a community-based intervention with sensitive responsiveness to individual needs (Home Office, 1998).

'Influence'

The 'influence on policies affecting health' has always been the most controversial of the principles, partly because it seems so large in scope and partly because health visitors are, arguably, considered too unimportant in the hierarchy of the health service to be permitted to 'influence'. However, the opportunities for health visitors to influence policy may increase with community nurse representatives (albeit in the minority in relation to GPs) contributing to Primary Care Group management. Twinn and Cowley (1992) suggest that the term 'policy' might be interpreted as referring to a local strategy to render it more manageable and less threatening. This formulation makes it possible to see much community development work as overlapping into this 'influencing' sphere of activity. Compiling community profiles for the purpose of influencing and advocating for more equitable service provision might, similarly, be regarded as an appropriate means of influencing strategies.

Cowley and Billings (1997), for example, used this approach to convince local health commissioners to invest in a full-time community development worker in one deprived area. Also, Alexander and McLean (1998) carried out a survey that revealed poor access to health care by travelling families; these authors convinced their local health authority of the importance of making special arrangements for this vulnerable group. However, there is little published research overall to either counter or support the wealth of anecdotal evidence that practitioners are often prevented from initiating the influence on policies affecting health.

'Stimulation'

The need for the population served to be aware of their own health needs is repeatedly stressed in health policy. A victim-blaming approach that implied fecklessness on the part of anyone who failed to adopt 'healthy behaviour' was stressed under the health policy of the former government's 'Health of the Nation' strategy (DoH, 1992). This has given way to a shared responsibility under recent proposals (DoH, 1998) stressing the important role of governments, local communities (including businesses and health services) and individuals. The need for a similar breadth was stressed by Twinn and Cowley (1992) when the principle of a 'stimulation of an awareness of health needs' was re-examined.

Cowley's (1991) qualitative research showed that considerable care is needed to negotiate the levels of awareness with clients, and with managers who did not always approve of the visiting aims and priorities agreed between practitioners and their clients. The abstract 'awareness context' within which these interactions take place may be conceptualised as reflecting all the social structures, preconceived prejudices and inequalities of society. Levels of awareness may be influenced by a strongly held belief or deep knowledge as well as the opposite – perhaps ignorance or a determined rejection or refusal even to acknowledge other people's perceptions or one's own position. This complexity accounts for some of the diversity of views on what constitutes a 'need' and fuels debate about how the service is best delivered.

The universal nature of the health visiting service, for example, seems important in enabling clients to see it as non-stigmatising (Orr, 1980; Mayall and Foster, 1989) and socially acceptable (see Chapter 6). However, from an organisational perspective, it can seem expensive and inefficient, so visiting all families with children under school age has been criticised for apparently failing to target needs effectively (Audit Commission, 1994; Roberts *et al.*, 1996). As suggested at the start of this chapter, these criticisms are based on the assumption that the health visiting service is needed only if a 'problem' already exists and that parents will identify their own health needs and seek help as required. These assumptions are not grounded in research; indeed, the opposite is more likely to be the case.

The universal child health promotion programme (Hall, 1996), for example, is recognised as an important opportunity for stimulating an awareness of health needs. This programme was promoted following a detailed review of research on child development; it provides the gateway to health needs assessment and increased levels of intervention by health service personnel (Appleton and Clemerson, 1999). It is considered important precisely because families may not easily reach the point at which they are able openly to acknowledge their half-formed worries or make any connection between their concerns and health – let alone health care. The offer of a focused opportunity to discuss their child acts as an acceptable mechanism and opportunity for discussing wider issues, which may lead on to apparently unrelated or hidden family health concerns (Collinson and Cowley, 1998a). Once a full awareness of health needs has been reached, practitioners can work in partnership with clients to find acceptable and practical solutions.

'Search'

This partnership approach is emphasised in the health visiting processes described by de la Cuesta (1993) and

Chalmers (1993). Chalmers showed that the skills utilised within the search for health needs varied from one situation to another. It could be initiated by clients as well as health visitors, and different approaches were used if the needs were easily seen or hidden. The health visitors described the need to implement skilful questioning, using examples from other client situations and responding to cues, even if those were hidden and hard to articulate. Furthermore, de la Cuesta (1993) described the way in which health visitors undertook 'fringe work' – activities that lay outside the official remit of their contract – in order to maintain a basis for work that was acceptable to their clients.

The apparent determination of some health commissioners to limit the scope of health visiting contradicts a well-recognised function of the role, in case-finding children 'in need' and their families (DoH, 1989, 1995). However, this key feature of the 'search for health needs' gives rise to criticisms that it has connotations of intrusiveness, suspicion and inspectorial attitudes. Abbott and Sapsford (1990), for example, accuse health visitors of adding to the difficulties that are already faced by mothers with young children by imposing unwelcome and judgemental attentions onto this group.

Where they exist, such negative attitudes undoubtedly have the potential to cause great harm. Families interviewed by Cowley and Billings (1999), for example, revealed that they encountered such negativity across a wide spectrum of health and welfare services; coping with this unpleasantness created stresses that, at times, outweighed the original need. However, health visitors acknowledge a professional responsibility to search for both recognised and unrecognised health needs in individuals, families and the wider community (CETHV, 1977). There will inevitably be competing agendas within some families and groups, and meeting these contradictory demands without causing offence requires considerable skill.

The health visitors interviewed by Cowley (1991) and Appleton (1994, 1995) generally revealed a strong personal sense of the need to approach sensitive and complex areas of need with great care, and actively to avoid intrusion and imposition. However, this was not easy in practice, particularly where the welfare of a child or vulnerable older person was a matter of concern. Indeed, the structured, controlling approach used in conversation by some health visitors has been strongly criticised for inhibiting participation (Kendall, 1993). Conversely, Dingwall and Robinson (1993) drew on a similar conversational analysis method to suggest that, in some circumstances, this approach is highly efficient and perceived as generally acceptable to the families being visited. They point out that, for the sake of children, society has a need to 'police' families, to expose hidden cases of serious abuse.

The conversational methods used by health visitors generally seem very successful in ensuring that children are protected without unduly interfering or compromising their parents. There is little overt acknowledgement of the surveillance role, but it is something of an 'open secret' (Dingwall, 1982). Furthermore, there is some evidence that families approve of this 'checking-up' role in certain circumstances. An unexpected enquiry that expresses personal interest and concern may be experienced as positive and caring (Collinson and Cowley, 1998b), for example. The key seems to lie not in the proactive nature of the enquiry but in the ability of the health visitor to convey a caring, interested stance rather than a judgemental and inquisitorial attitude.

The search for health needs

This volume brings together a collection of health visiting research that adds to this knowledge of how health visitors search for health needs. None of the studies began with the overt intention of exploring this aspect of health visiting practice, but each adds to the collective understanding of the complex, contested nature of the principle.

The assumption that health needs exist only in the presence of an established problem is challenged by the focus taken by Cowley in Chapter 2. This explains how health visitors tend to treat health as process, which requires the use and development of positive 'resources for health'. Instead of targeting problems (and creating stigmatised 'problem people'), this allows need to be conceptualised as existing within the wider situation. This positive focus contradicts the usual approach within the NHS, which has traditionally tended to focus on negative disease-orientated concerns. The dilemmas of utilising such an approach are contrasted with the swift returns required by short-term contract arrangements for community health services and the demand for rapid outcome measures. In Chapter 8, Kelsey explores the difficulties faced by health visiting as it strives to reach a way of identifying outcome measures that do not compromise the underlying values of the profession.

In Chapter 3, Twinn examines some of the complexities that are involved in practitioners making assessments of families' health needs. Coming from an educational perspective, it debates the skills and knowledge required for this work, pointing to the importance of professional artistry and a depth of reflective ability for practice. As well as considering how the identification of health needs may be informed by professional judgement, the use of guidelines to prioritise family needs is also addressed. The past decade has seen considerable interest in the development of clinical practice guidelines and protocols in the health service to facilitate practitioners in the process of needs assessment. In Chapter 4, Appleton assesses the extent to which clinical guidelines are issued to health visitors to assist in the identification of families requiring increased interventions and to examine their validity and reliability.

Realistically, the identification of health and social need by community nurses cannot be undertaken in isolation. Indeed, this type of work must be carried out in conjunction with clients, community groups, residents, activists and advocates such as voluntary organisations and other members of the primary health care team. Machin, in Chapter 6, emphasises the importance of health visitors providing a service that is acceptable to mothers and reflects their expressed needs. The dilemmas encountered in ensuring that consumer perceptions of health needs are represented accurately and that they are given equal voice are explored by Billings in Chapter 5 and Blackburn in Chapter 7. These studies examine how consumers' perceptions of their own health needs and their health visiting service may be used to inform practice.

Overall, this volume has been written with the intention of disseminating some of this research work to a wider audience. Its focus on the health visiting search for health needs is intended to make research findings more accessible for community practitioners; the authors have identified a few key points at the end of each chapter. Health and health needs assessment are recognised as the foundation for preventive work and ensuing health care endeavours. The book has attempted to collect together recent research relevant to the identification of health needs at both an individual and a population level, and all chapters examine the complex relationship between health visiting and the identification of health needs. However, it is presumed that much of the information in this book will be applicable and of potential interest to groups other than health visitors who, like them, are involved in primary prevention.

Contributions have been sought that provide some insight into a broad range of different research approaches. The chapters are written by the original researchers, who report on their chosen methodology and reflect on the implications of their work for community nursing practice, education or policy. It is hoped that this will encourage readers to consider ways to improve the 'search for health needs', whether this is carried out as an assessment or identification of health needs, for planning or for implementing services directed at health promotion and preventive health care. Finally, it is hoped that the volume will stimulate further discussion and research to add to the dynamic and growing body of knowledge in community nursing and health visiting.

KEY POINTS

■ Health need is a complex concept that has come to the fore of health policy since the implementation of the NHS and Community Care Act 1990.
However, health visitors recognised the importance of searching out both
acknowledged and unacknowledged health needs long before that legislation was implemented.

■ Competing views about what constitutes a legitimate 'health need' influence service planning and provision. The idea that health needs consist
only of problems or diseases that are amenable to treatment is highly
influential; this definition is unhelpful in determining the nature of health
needs to be targeted by health-promoting services.

■ Health visitors have a history of clarifying and articulating their knowledge base through working groups. In this way, the principles of health
visiting, which include the idea of the 'search for health needs', were initially identified. This approach is giving way to a more sophisticated,
research-based means of developing their professional knowledge.

■ This collection of studies that are relevant to the search for health needs
is offered to stimulate discussion and further research, as well as to
provide a basis to guide and inform practice.

References

Abbott P. and Sapsford R. (1990) Health visiting: policing the family?
In Abbott P. and Wallace C. (eds) *The Sociology of the Caring Professions*. Basingstoke: Falmer Press.

Alexander S. and Mclean C. (1998) Report for the Pilot Health
Promotion Project with Travellers in Dorset. Glastonbury: Friends,
Families and Travellers Support Group.

Angeli N. (1994) Facilitating parenting skills in vulnerable families.
Health Visitor **67**(4): 130–2.

Appleton J.V. (1994) The concept of vulnerability in relation to
child protection: health visitors' perceptions. *Journal of Advanced
Nursing* **20**(6): 1132–40.

Appleton J.V. (1995) Health visitor assessment of vulnerability. *Health
Visitor* **68**(6): 228–31.

Appleton J.V. (1996) Working with vulnerable families: a health
visiting perspective. *Journal of Advanced Nursing* **23**: 912–18.

Appleton J.V. and Clemerson J. (1999) Issues for staff in health. In
Calder M.C. and Horwath J. (eds) *Working for Children on the Child*

Protection Register: An Inter-agency Practice Guide. Aldershot: Arena (in press).

Ashton J. and Seymour H. (1988) *The New Public Health.* Milton Keynes: Open University Press.

Audit Commission (1994) *Seen but not Heard: Co-ordinating Community Child Health and Social Services for Children in Need.* London: HMSO.

Bergen A., Cowley S., Young K. and Kavanagh A. (1996) *An Investigation into the Changing Educational Needs of Community Nurses with Regard to Needs Assessment and Quality of Care in the Context of the NHS and Community Care Act, 1990.* London: English National Board for Nursing, Midwifery and Health Visiting.

Billings J. and Cowley S. (1995) Approaches to community needs assessment: a literature review. *Journal of Advanced Nursing* **22**: 721–30.

Boyd M., Brummell K., Billingham K. and Perkins E. (1993) *The Public Health Post at Strelley: An Interim Report.* Nottingham: Nottingham Community Health Trust.

Brown I. (1997) A skill mix parent support initiative in health visiting: an evaluation study. *Health Visitor* **70**(9): 339–43.

Buchan H., Gary M., Hill A. and Coulter A. (1990) Needs assessment made simple. *Health Service Journal* (15 Feb): 240–1.

Campbell F., Cowley S. and Buttigieg M. (1995) *Weights and Measures: Outcomes and Evaluation in Health Visiting.* London: Health Visitors' Association.

Carney O., McIntosh J., Worth A. and Lugton J. (1996) *Assessment of Need for Health Visiting Department of Nursing and Community Health.* Glasgow: Glasgow Caledonian University.

Chalmers K. (1993) Searching for health needs: the work of health visiting. *Journal of Advanced Nursing* **18**(6): 900–11.

Clough D. (1980) Conference paper reported in *The Investigation Debate: A Commentary on An Investigation into the Principles of Health Visiting.* London: CETHV.

Collinson S. and Cowley S. (1998a) Exploring need: taking the marketing perspective. *Community Practitioner* **71**: 244–7.

Collinson S. and Cowley S. (1998b) An exploratory study of demand for the health visiting service, within a marketing framework. *Journal of Advanced Nursing* **28**: 499–507.

Colver A.F., Hutchinson P.J. and Judson E.C. (1982) Promoting children's home safety. *British Medical Journal* **285**: 1177–80.

Coombes G. (1991) *You Can't Watch Them 24 Hours a Day.* London: Child Accident Prevention Trust.

Council for the Education and Training of Health Visitors (CETHV) (1977) *An Investigation into the Principles of Health Visiting.* London:

CETHV (reprinted 1993, English National Board for Nursing, Midwifery and Health Visiting, London).

Council for the Education and Training of Health Visitors (CETHV) (1980) *The Investigation Debate: A Commentary on an Investigation into the Principles of Health Visiting.* London: CETHV.

Council for the Education and Training of Health Visitors (CETHV) (1982) *Principles in Practice.* London: CETHV.

Cowley S. (1991) A symbolic awareness context identified through a grounded theory of health visiting. *Journal of Advanced Nursing* **16**: 648–56.

Cowley S. (1996) Reflecting on the past; preparing for the next century. *Health Visitor* **69**(8): 313–16.

Cowley S. (1997) Public health values in practice: the case of health visiting. *Critical Public Health* **7**: 82–97.

Cowley S. and Billings J. (1997) *Family Health Needs Project.* Research Report; South Thames Primary Care Development Fund, London: Department of Nursing Studies, King's College, London.

Cowley S. and Billings J. (1999) Resources revisited: salutogenesis from a lay perspective. *Journal of Advanced Nursing* **20**: 994–1004.

Craig P. (1996) Drumming up health in Drumchapel: community development health visiting. *Health Visitor* **69**(11): 460–2.

Crew K. and Fletcher J. (1995) Empowering parents to prevent childhood accidents. *Health Visitor* **68**(7): 291.

Cuesta C. de la (1993) Fringe work: peripheral work in health visiting. *Sociology of Health and Illness* **15**(5): 667–82.

Davies C. (1988) The health visitor as mother's friend: a woman's place in public health, 1900–1914. *Social History of Medicine* **1**(1): 39–59.

Davis H., Spurr P., Cox A., Lynch M., von Roenne A. and Hahn K. (1997) A description and evaluation of a community child mental health service. *Clinical Child Psychology and Psychiatry* **2**(2): 221–38.

Department of Health (DoH) (1989) *Working for Patients.* Cmnd 555. London: HMSO.

Department of Health (DoH) (1992) *The Health of the Nation: A Strategy for Health in England.* London: HMSO.

Department of Health (DoH) (1995) *Child Protection: Messages from Research.* London: HMSO.

Department of Health (DoH) (1997) *The New NHS: Modern, Dependable.* Cmnd 3809. London: Stationery Office.

Department of Health (DoH) (1998) *Our Healthier Nation: A Contract for Health.* Cmnd 3852. London: Stationery Office.

Dingwall R. (1977) Collectivism, regionalism and feminism: health visiting and British social policy. *Journal of Social Policy* **6**(3): 291–315.

Dingwall R. (1982) Community nursing and civil liberty. *Journal of Advanced Nursing* **7**: 337–46.

Dingwall R. and Robinson K. (1993) Policing the family? Health visiting and the public surveillance of private behaviour. In Beattie A., Gott M., Jones L. and Sidell M. (eds) *Health and Well-being: A Reader*. Basingstoke: Macmillan.

Edwards J. (1995) 'Parenting skills': views of community health and social service providers about the needs of their 'clients'. *Journal of Social Policy* **24**: 237–59.

Edwards J. and Popay J. (1994) Contradictions of support and self-help: views from providers of community health and social services to families with young children. *Health and Social Care in the Community* **2**(1): 31–40.

Hall D. (1996) *Health for All Children*, (3rd edn). Oxford: Oxford University Press.

Health Service Circular (HSC) Review of the Nurses, Midwives and Health Visitors Act: Government response to the recommendations DOH, HSC 1999/030.

Home Office (1988) *Supporting Families: A Consultation Document*. London: Stationery Office.

J.M. Consulting (1998) *The Regulation of Nurses, Midwives and Health Visitors*. Bristol: J.M. Consulting.

Kendall S. (1993) Do health visitors promote client participation? An analysis of the health visitor–client interaction. *Journal of Clinical Nursing* **2**: 103–9.

Kerr S., Jowett S. and Smith L. (1997) Education to help prevent sleep problems in infants. *Health Visitor* **70**(6): 224–5.

Mackereth C. (1997) Health visiting: is it a nursing matter? *Health Visitor* **70**(4): 155–7.

Mayall B. and Foster M.-C. (1989) *Child Health Care: Living with Children, Working for Children*. Oxford: Heinemann Nursing.

NHS Executive (NHSE) (1996) *Child Health in the Community: A Guide to Good Practice*. London: DoH.

Orr J. (1980) *Health Visiting in Focus*. London: RCN.

Orr J. (1992) Assessing individual and family health needs. In Luker K. and Orr J. (eds) *Health Visiting: Towards Community Health Nursing*, (2nd edn). Oxford: Blackwell Scientific.

Pearson P. (1991) Clients' perceptions: the use of case studies in developing theory. *Journal of Advanced Nursing* **16**: 521–8.

Pritchard P. (1994) Behavioural work with pre-school children in the community. *Health Visitor* **67**(2): 54–6.

Rees-Jones I. (1995) Health care need and contracts for health services. *Health Care Analysis* **3**: 91–8.

Roberts H., Smith S. and Bryce C. (1993) Prevention is better... *Sociology of Health and Illness* **16**(4): 447–63.

Roberts I., Kramer M. and Suissa S. (1996) Does home visiting prevent childhood injury? A systematic review of randomised controlled trials. *British Medical Journal* **312**: 29–33.

Robinson J. (1982) *An Evaluation of Health Visiting.* London: CETHV.

Robinson J. (1985) Health visiting and health: political issues. In White R. (ed.) *Nursing: Past, Present and Future.* Chichester: John Wiley & Sons.

Rowbotham A. (1998) Health visiting education: challenging present systems. *Community Practitioner* **71**: 215–18.

Standing Nursing and Midwifery Advisory Committee (SNMAC) (1995) *Making it Happen. Public Health: The Contribution, Role and Development of Nurses, Midwives and Health Visitors.* London: DoH.

Stevens A. and Gabbay J. (1991) Needs assessment needs assessment. *Health Trends* **23**(1): 20–3.

Summers A. and McKeown K. (1996) Health needs assessment in primary care: a role for health visitors. *Health Visitor* **69**(8): 323–4.

Symonds A. (1997) Medical mantras: why health visiting risks losing its way. *Health Visitor* **70**(3): 99–100.

Twinn S. (1991) Conflicting paradigms of health visiting: a continuing debate for practice. *Journal of Advanced Nursing* **16**: 966–73.

Twinn S. (1993) Principles in practice: a re-affirmation. *Health Visitor* **66**(9): 319–21.

Twinn S. and Cowley S. (1992) *The Principles of Health Visiting: A Re-examination.* London: HVA/United Kingdom Standing Conference.

United Kingdom Central Council for Nursing, Midwifery and Health Visiting (UKCC) (1994) *The Future of Professional Practice – The Council's Standards for Education and Practice Following Registration.* London: UKCC.

United Kingdom Central Council for Nursing, Midwifery and Health Visiting (UKCC) (1998) *Standards for Specialist Education and Practice.* London: UKCC.

2

Situation and Process in Health Visiting

Sarah Cowley

Despite increasing legislative emphasis on the idea of assessing health needs prior to planning or delivering services (DoH, 1989, 1997), policy details neither specify what counts as a 'need' nor how it should be defined. There is a dearth of information about how 'health needs' should be specified in relation to health promotion within the well population, in whom no actual change in individual health status is sought. Without such information, the assumption that health is the absence of disease has underpinned successive health service policies, including those specifically concerned with health promotion.

This is particularly relevant to service definitions and functions carried out by health visitors, whose practice consists of planned activities aimed at the promotion of health (CETHV, 1977). If need is construed as the presence of a disease or (at least) of a problem that is amenable to change by health service intervention, only individuals with specified illnesses or risks are viewed as a legitimate focus for attention in a 'needs-led' health service. In such formulations, the well population is perceived as having no potential to benefit from clinical interventions; this leads to the further assumption that they have no general need for a health-promoting service and thus no need for health visiting on a regular or routine basis (NHSE, 1996).

Indeed, although the health visitors' function has always been specifically concerned with health promotion, health visiting work can appear unfocused, diffuse, difficult to explain and often contrary to prevailing policies. In the light of this, there has been an upsurge in research by health visitors since the early 1980s, with an emphasis on explaining both the process and the outcome of the work. Several studies, including the one reported in this chapter, have aimed to illuminate the processes and hidden features embedded within health visiting practice using a grounded theory approach (for example Pearson, 1991; Chalmers, 1992, 1994; de la Cuesta, 1993, 1994). The study reported here revealed how, in the absence of a need for clinical intervention, health visitors appeared to assess needs by treating health as a process fuelled by the accumulation and use of 'resources for health'.

Situation and process

The study reported here used grounded theory to examine how health visitors select an approach to use in any particular situation; some aspects of the analysis appear elsewhere (Cowley, 1991, 1995a, 1995b). It revealed a way of treating health that is internally consistent but potentially at odds with the disease-led policies that control NHS spending and service planning.

Grounded theory

Grounded theory is a strategy for handling data in research that aims to 'capture the complexity of reality... and... make convincing sense of it' (Strauss, 1987: 10). It is an approach that is recommended when little is known about the field of study (Glaser and Strauss, 1967; Glaser, 1978) or to gain a fresh perspective in a familiar situation (Stern, 1985). The aim is to generate a new theory, which is a form of explanation, that is 'grounded' firmly in the field from which the data are drawn; it is not concerned with validating or testing existing theories. Three important features are present together in grounded theory: theoretical sampling, constant comparative analysis and theoretical saturation. Each of these may occur separately in other forms of qualitative research but all three are required to ensure that the grounded theory is validated as it is discovered through these processes.

Theoretical sampling involves the concurrent collection, coding and analysis of data as a matrix procedure rather than a linear operation. The eventual form of the theory is unknown at the outset, so neither the eventual sample nor the exact questions can be predicted in advance. Data are analysed as they are collected, and the ideas, hunches and themes that emerge from the analysis are used to inform decisions about where and how to collect the next tranche of data. Using this approach, data were gathered from 53 practising health visitors, mainly through a series of informal small group interviews, but also through observation in baby clinics and discussions about tape-recorded home visits. The health visitors were all female; they were volunteers, drawn from refresher courses run by the Health Visitors' Association that recruit nationally, from one course of preparation for community practice teachers and from two separate employing authorities in the South East of England.

The process known as constant comparative analysis involves breaking the data into minute fragments and examining them from multiple different angles, much as one might view various slices, wedges or sections of a microscopic specimen to discover a full picture of how the item is constructed. The aim is to abstract raw concepts from the data in order to encourage theorising and sensitivity to the field from which the data were drawn. Altogether, 1003 separate fragments of data were indexed onto separate cards, each containing up to five separate concepts and theoretical notes. In the interests of auditability (Guba and Lincoln, 1985), each concept could be traced back to the data from which it was first elicited. The concepts that come directly from the data are intended to yield a full, rich description of the substantive field from which they are drawn. Concepts elicited in the analysis are used in wording the final report to demonstrate the authenticity and 'grounding' of the emergent theory in the data.

Following Glaser (1978), these diverse concepts were gradually aggregated under higher-order, complex concepts, sometimes known as 'categories', adding richness and meaning to the emerging theory. Literature is treated as data; instead of the standard literature review at the start of the report, therefore, excerpts and insights from relevant studies are integrated into the analysis and theory as it emerges. Notes were kept of the concepts, hunches and working hypotheses generated throughout the analytic process and a search was made for recurring themes and uniformities. These are the 'theoretical codes' that eventually lead to the formulation of the conceptual framework that structures the grounded theory. Throughout the analysis, a search is made for a 'core concept', which is a significant higher-order process or dimension that can account for most of the variation in the data.

Eventually, when the joint procedures of data collection and analysis provide no new insights, a point of 'theoretical saturation' is reached and the process is deemed complete. This chapter summarises the concept of health encapsulated in the analysis and considers how this formulation could be used more explicitly to determine the scope and focus of health visiting interactions.

Health as process

The idea of treating health as a process was identified as a higher-order concept in this study. Once this had been identified, it became possible to integrate many other less complex concepts into a unifying theoretical framework based upon it. These included a number of factors, summarised in Table 2.1, that would otherwise appear to be unrelated. The theory suggests these factors need taking into account in decisions of what type of health visiting approach to use in any particular situation.

The analysis suggested that, by treating health as a process, health visitors could integrate a number of competing and alternative views and beliefs about health into a single perspective or framework upon which to base their practice. The idea of health as a process is entirely abstract; it is not observable, but it can be conceptualised. The concept was not consciously expressed in the data, but the idea recurred throughout the health visitors' descriptions of their practice and perceptions of health.

An international review of health promotion practices and concepts identified that health may be viewed in one of three ways (Anderson, 1984). In the traditional medical formulation, health is viewed as a 'product', bound up with notions of disease. It may also be viewed as 'potential'; Seedhouse (1986) is perhaps most often associated with the idea that positive health is a means by which opportunities of life can be realised.

Table 2.1 Factors affecting health visiting

Health	Health visiting approaches
Health needs defined by:	Assessment through:
• resource availability in situation • position of individual in context • problem/illness: present or predicted (risk factors)	• experiential knowledge • lay perspectives • empirical knowledge • normative criteria
Direction of health-as-process?	Respond to direction of process:
• positive • turning point • negative	• promote positive development • therapeutic prevention • crisis intervention
Level?	Promote resources for health:
• individual • family • community/group	• caring/therapeutic approaches • educational approaches

The idea of health as a process is the third concept identified by Anderson. This concept of health emphasises (Anderson, 1984: 61):

an ever changing, dynamic phenomenon or process... [which]... may relate to optimum physical growth and body development. The health process may be cumulative in relation, for example, to learning and development or cyclical in phases of creation and destruction. The point appears to be that health is a continuing pattern of change occurring over the lifetime in all dimensions of the individual.

Although this is similar to the idea of health as 'potential', a key difference lies in the fact that 'processes' require context and meaning to make sense of them, so linkages, patterns, interconnections and actions are emphasised more than separate factors or events. If health is viewed as a process, it is not possible to conceive of any aspect of it that can stand alone or be under the control of anyone other than the people whose health is under discussion: the whole sociocultural context is important. In this formulation, a holistic emphasis includes not only the whole individual, but also the whole environment and situation in which people live.

Stages in the process

In any process, change occurs over time, and there are at least two clearly demarcated stages, transitional states that have a beginning and an end (Glaser, 1978). The states of illness and well-being (and the huge diversity of understanding encompassed within these concepts) can be viewed as transitional stages in the process of health. Conceptually, this makes it possible to separate health care actions directed at realising and promoting the continuing and cumulative processes of health from activities directed at changing the separate stages of illness or well-being. Both of these states can be recognised by the person experiencing them, or by an outside observer using empirical, scientific knowledge, but the two perceptions may differ. A person may feel well but may have a hidden disease process detectable on examination, for example a malignant change in the cervix; alternatively, a person feeling unwell may have no discernible medical signs or symptoms despite being subjectively in a state of illness.

Kolb (1984) promotes the idea of a dual knowledge theory in which information gained through sensation (that is, direct apprehension) is just as important as comprehension, that is, the rational, empirical form of knowing. Similarly, the data in this study suggested that, on the whole, the health visitors understood and accepted the scientific and medical explanations for health and illness but wished to value the subjective experience of their clients and their own professional judgements, sometimes above that normative information.

However, the work situation sometimes constrained health visitors into giving priority to organisationally defined, normative needs. Lay perspectives may be appropriate and useful when defining the needs to be targeted; indeed, a number of practitioners claimed that they deferred to these views in private while presenting the 'public face' of using the professionally accepted terminology and targets when reporting to their managers. A key requirement of health visiting appears to be an ability to understand and value both the 'private face' and hidden health needs experienced within families and the explicit accountability required in a publicly financed health service, as well as the skill to work across the interface between public and private spheres.

The analysis suggested that the health visitors largely directed their attention towards the processes and associated context rather than only focusing on the states of illness or well-being. The need for input seemed to be assessed according to the possibility of a negative transition in the dynamic health process rather than the exact nature of the particular, specified or undesirable health state.

Resources for health

The grounded theory offers a hypothetical explanation for transition or change in the process in terms of the accumulation and use of positive elements that might serve as 'resources for health'. These resources were not specified in any depth in the analysis as no data were drawn from the clients themselves. The resources appeared to be personal and situational rather than being specifically limited to consumer items or financial means, although such resources as good housing and adequate income are clearly important for health. Resources for health appeared infinitely variable, being potentially internalised, individual and personal, or possibly arising from the situation in which the clients lived. Personal examples included emotional resources such as self-esteem, a sense of trust in self and others (perhaps a partner or family), physical stamina or the cognitive ability to learn how to cope with a new baby. Situational resources might arise from the local environment, community and cultural influences at a wider level or be drawn from formally provided services.

The health visitors explained that they needed to be aware of their clients' potential for developing and accumulating resources for health. For a variety of reasons, some people may be unable to envisage their own potential or fully understand what health might mean to them:

> sometimes you can see things that are possible for them [clients] that they can't see. It's not that you would choose for them, because it must be up to them, but people don't always know, or make the connections, so it's up to you as a health visitor to let them know. (HV2)

Such views link personal development and health, implying that health is conceived of as a process that is integral to the individual rather than a product that can exist independently of the person. The data suggested that some health visitors recognised the need for a certain amount of 'consciousness-raising' or 'emancipatory education' of the kind envisaged by community educationalists such as Freire (1970) and Mezirow (1981). The process may be quite similar to the ideas embedded in the health visiting principle of the 'stimulation of the awareness of health needs' (CETHV, 1977: 9). This humanistic educational approach was widely favoured when the health visitors were considering situations in which no immediate threats to health were identified, but it was also used to help people to avoid specific, identifiable risks.

When resources for health seemed in short supply, or when negative influences prevailed, an explicitly caring approach was favoured. The word 'care' appeared very little in the data, but many comments conveyed an impression of a strong emotional commitment towards the client or group. Examples of concepts that emerged from the analysis and that might demonstrate care included 'giving time' even when busy, 'fitting the service to the need' in a way that personalised it, 'being with' someone in times of stress and staying in contact with people who had, perhaps, been rejected or dismissed by other professional services, their families or friends. Terms drawn from humanistic counselling such as 'support' and 'relationship' were common, for example:

> It needs a human being to give her [the client] some support and show that we care, that we're going to listen even if we haven't got a magic formula to listen... You just give her the support that she is doing all right. (HV48)

The potential variety of interacting resources appeared so great that each combination needed to be viewed as unique to the individual and to the situation in which the person was living. However, noting whether or not resources were present or positive seemed to be an important part of a health visiting assessment of where needs might lie.

Health at many levels

Health can potentially be experienced at many different levels – from the microscopic, cellular level through the whole organism of an individual person, to groups, localities and countries, possibly even to the whole planet. It is thus considered to be as reasonable to talk in terms of a 'healthy city' (WHO, 1986) as it is to conclude from a cellular examination that someone has a 'healthy cervix'.

The data indicated that the health visitors did not plan to work only at a microscopic level, the health of a whole person representing the outer limits of their responsibility.

Nor did they seem to centre, epidemiologically, on population groups so large as to obscure individual variation or statistically insignificant pockets of deprivation. Instead, they focused their attention mainly at the interface where individuals, families and groups meet and interact. The data implied that both educational and caring interventions could be targeted at the multiple levels, so a family, a whole community or an identified group of people might learn collectively or develop new capacities, or be offered and experience support, for example. Treating health as a process that evolves through interactions at multiple levels and in many dimensions may help to stabilise the apparently confusing diversity of this interface so that it becomes more manageable. It is also a potentially efficient way of developing resources that might contribute to health across families or communities.

An assessment of the level – individual or group – from which possible threats to well-being may arise, or from which potential resources for health may be drawn, incorporates a breadth that seemed important to the health visitors in this study. The data indicated several examples to show how health visitors might shift the focus of their assessment or intervention from an individual to a wider, collective level. One health visitor working in the Channel Islands considered the needs of a caseload that was sometimes transient as families from the mainland accompanied partners seconded by employers for a period of time:

> There were no mother and toddler groups on the island, and we were identifying that there were a lot of mums who were particularly isolated – maybe mothers who were going to be over here for a short space of time – things like banks – they're only here for two or three years. They didn't have any extended family on the island and they needed to know other people, so the idea was put into the mothers' heads about the idea of mother and toddler groups with the idea of the parents starting one themselves which they did do. (HV34)

There are two incidental issues encapsulated in this excerpt. The first is the very long timespan over which health visiting appears to operate. Health as a process is a lifelong concept; 'two or three or years' seems a remarkably short space of time when placed in that context, but such an outlook contravenes the rapid throughput, short-term contracts and calls for annual measures of health-related outcomes that prevail within the current NHS. Second, the idea of 'putting an idea into the mothers' heads' emphasises the point that health visiting is rarely about 'doing things for people'; descriptive concepts elicited from the data emphasise that it more usually proceeds by 'facil-itation', by 'being a catalyst', by 'suggesting' or 'hinting', or by 'getting (things or clients) started'.

Types of health visiting input

Broadly speaking, the types of intervention explained by the health visitors could generally be regarded as either educational or caring in intent. The former were not restricted to traditional health education methods but incorporated broad approaches to development at a community, group or individual level. Caring approaches derived from the therapeutic endeavour of nursing or humanistic psychology; again, these might be directed at individuals, whole families or wider groups.

A further distinction in the type of activity was closely linked to the central theme of treating health as a process. This abstract idea can explain how health visitors respond to the possibility of a negative transition in the process itself rather than to the exact nature of a particular, spec-ified and undesirable health state to which it may lead. The timing and type of input seem to relate to the expected speed at which a transition may occur. Three alternative activities were detailed:

- crisis intervention
- therapeutic prevention
- promoting positive development.

'Crisis interventions' seemed to be activated in rapidly changing situations when an adverse event or problem was either imminent or had already occurred. The metaphorical health process would be negative in direction, so interventions would be directed at halting its downward trajectory. The notion of 'crisis' was invoked in the data when an immediate response was required, even if it meant pushing other activities to one side. This sense of immediacy seemed to be the defining feature since the term did not appear to indicate severity. As one health visitor explained:

> Yes, we're still the crisis visitors, just the same way as the district nurses. It can be somebody – an elderly person who's already tripped over the rug and broken a leg and perhaps needs a walking stick... (HV48)

In this approach, routes to health promotion often remained unclear, except perhaps by analogy with the tertiary prevention of disease, but the starting points were immediately apparent. Geissler (1984) notes that the cause of a crisis is likely to be specific but the effect non-specific. In the present study, numerous specific events were identified that would lead to crisis visiting: maternal illness, child abuse, postnatal depression, accidents, hospitalisation and so on. Most of the health visitors expressed a degree of resignation, accepting crisis work as a necessary, if unwelcome, part of their role. However, if it came to predominate as a way of working, new ways of thinking about how to deliver services were required:

> We did health visiting priorities in... because we were all doing crisis visiting and we were all so demoralised because that's not health visiting, just crisis visiting. (HV38)

The interventions were characterised by offering help, direct advice or care that could have an immediate, if short-lived, impact. The idea was to bring clients through the current difficulty so that they could reach a point at which they could resume constructing their own decisions and solutions. Because of the immediate need for health-related resources, the generation of 'spare' resources through learning or personal development is not a priority in crisis intervention.

However, if a family is overwhelmed by ongoing difficulties, perhaps with limited personal resources and little to call upon from the wider situation within which they live, a kind of 'continuing crisis' is likely to arise, and some way of breaking the cycle is needed. One way of achieving this is to shift attention to a wider level of health, concentrating on the local community rather than the individual. This will also help if there are a number of such families in a local area, when a single caseload may be dominated by the need for crisis work. Formal services will inevitably be stretched by increasing calls upon them as 'proxy' resources for health if no responses are directed at creating new capacity. Concentrating on crisis intervention was generally regarded as a kind of failure by the health visitors because it was considered counterproductive to health across the wider arena.

At the opposite extreme, a person or family may have sufficient resources for health within their own situation. In such circumstances, the direction of health-as-process could remain positive despite a specific trauma or difficulty, or even in the face of multiple challenges such as those encountered by people with long-term disabilities. If there is no immediate threat to a specified individual's health, the idea of focusing on resources within a situation can be more helpful than concentrating on 'problems'. This can overcome the difficult question of establishing who, within a family, 'owns' a particular need or problem, for example:

> with things like sleep problems – the child is thriving and is healthy and looks perfectly OK but wants to stay up all night. The problem isn't the baby's – it's the parents'... because some families will have a baby that stays up all night and that's fine, but if that baby happens to be in a different household who feel they need a regular routine that's really a problem, sort of a mismatch. (HV9)

Dealing with such matters involves the use of certain health-related resources, perhaps patience, understanding, stamina or an ability to set immediate requirements into a meaningful context. However, even if the demand for such resources is high, a positive direction in the process of health can be sustained as long as resources can be actively renewed and regenerated. Health visiting interventions in such situations will focus on promoting positive development, being broadly educational in intent and focused on the wider situation or context rather than on a specific problem. In view of this, there may be no specific change identifiable in the individual (although one may occur), but enhancing the resources for health across a whole area or caseload could, presumably, contribute to a change in the wider situation.

Because both the approaches and the situations that require them are so different, the health visiting activities directed at promoting positive development or at crisis intervention were generally mutually exclusive. However, a third type of intervention was identified – 'therapeutic prevention', lying between the other two types in terms of urgency. This intervention appears both common in practice and distinctively associated with health visiting. It focused on the wider situational context for families with multiple difficulties that were poorly specified but nevertheless distressing.

The complexity embedded in the situations that elicited this type of intervention has been reported in detail elsewhere (Cowley, 1995b). The situations are distinguished by uncertainty and ambiguity: they are not clearly either normal or abnormal; they include an element of suffering and distress, and a risk that an abnormal situation may arise or an existing, hidden health problem be missed. The response of 'therapeutic prevention' is a complex blend of caring and educational interventions used when the direction of the health process is not yet clear. Considerable skill is required to implement the approach in order to hold the uncertainty within the situation while simultaneously targeting the suffering by offering a therapeutic 'caring' stance and providing education to avoid precipitating the risk of deterioration.

Although there is no specific disorder to avoid, the approach may be best viewed as analogous to secondary prevention. A number of health visitors expressed frustration that situations that were clearly urgent from their perspective were not regarded as such by non-health visiting colleagues. Using the notion of health as a process, it is possible to conceptualise these critical periods as potential turning points that require tremendous care to redirect. The importance of focusing on the whole context appears to be particularly significant in dealing with ambiguous and uncertain situations. It avoids the stigma associated with singling out individuals and prematurely labelling situations as abnormal. Furthermore, focusing on the whole situation rather than on an unclear and unspecified problem appears to be more fruitful in identifying solutions.

This grounded theory offers a tentative explanation and framework that might guide health visiting practice. The analysis does not, in itself, provide a basis for explaining how health is created; it offers only an explanation of how health visitors apparently treat health – an outlook that may or may not be justified. However, while grounded theory starts without a literature review, the 'fresh look' identified once the analysis is complete can guide searches of other relevant literature. There are some key areas of research that provide justification for a health visiting focus on context and process in the pursuit of health.

Salutogenesis

There is a view that health is directly opposite to disease, or that health is present when disease is absent. Accordingly, a great deal of practice and research aims to identify the causes and best treatments of specific diseases – that is the science of 'pathogenesis'. The opposite view assumes that health can exist even in the presence of disease or disability, and that the existence of risk factors does not mean that a disorder or dysfunction will inevitably result. This leads to the science of 'salutogenesis', which is concerned with identifying factors that create health rather than disease, and with exploring aspects that contribute to healing or to resistance to physiological or psychological breakdown.

The idea of salutogenesis is drawn from the philosophy and research of Antonovsky (1987), whose definition of health as a 'sense of coherence' provides a theoretical basis for explaining how health may be created. The reliability and validity of this concept have been widely tested and shown to be rigorous (Antonovsky, 1993). Life experiences are assumed to produce 'generalised resistance resources', which are positive methods of responding and adapting to situations. These resistance resources promote a pervasive, enduring and dynamic feeling of confidence that things will work out as well as can reasonably be expected. Being based in a personal 'sense of coherence' locates this theory very closely to the person's own context, expectations and culture, but it incorporates practical aspects as well. Antonovsky's research does not include a practice component, but the concepts incorporated in his theory are fully consistent with the idea of 'resources for health' used in analysing the health visiting data outlined above.

This salutogenic model shows how health may be created at an individual or family level, and it is clearly based within a social rather than a medical framework. Mechanisms by which this is translated into health across families or populations are less clear, but a growing literature suggests that social cohesion is an important determinant of health (Blane *et al.*, 1996; Wilkinson, 1996). This is closely aligned to the idea of 'social capital', which refers to the norms of reciprocity and networks of civic engagement. These become embedded and enacted through moral resources such as trust and co-operation across the whole social system rather than only by individuals (Putnam, 1993). Mustard (1996) links this idea with 'health capital' by identifying forces that influence health across populations, such as socioeconomic factors, childhood, competence and coping skills, and health service policies.

This theory also offers a salutogenic explanation by focusing on activities that build and create health rather than only on the destructive forces of disease; once more, the idea of the accumulation and use of 'resources' to influence and create health is considered. However, these resources must, apparently, be developed by the people concerned in order to be meaningful and useful. This was the lesson of a further study carried out by Cowley and Billings (1997, 1999), who analysed data drawn from the main care-taker – mainly the mother – in 50 families with resident preschool and school-aged children to elicit a lay perspective about how people create or maintain their own health. Aspects of this study are reported in Chapter 5 of this volume. Cowley and Billings' study demonstrated that the process of developing a capacity for resourcefulness in creating health, particularly in times of stress and hardship, was associated with the concept of personal empowerment.

Empowerment is a multilevel construct that applies to individual citizens or neighbourhoods; as Rappaport (1987) explains, it implies the study of people in context. The capacity to develop or use resources for health was shown on analysis to disseminate from an individual to a community or across generations, suggesting that this process may help contribute to the health and social capital of local areas and, in turn, the social cohesiveness and sustainability of health across a wider population. The importance of context and subjective experience in these lay descriptions of health creation draws attention to the need to identify ways of promoting health that are related to salutogenic rather than pathogenic processes.

Conclusion

This chapter reported a grounded theory that offers an internally consistent explanation of the way in which health visitors appear to assess needs with a view to promoting health. It suggests that they concentrate on the wider situation and context within which their clients live rather than focusing only on specified existing or potential problems or disorders. The study offered no insights into the way in which health is actually created, but it drew attention to other theories of salutogenesis, and to new research about social cohesion and health and social capital. Together, these provide a robust underpinning explanation of how health may be generated and maintained, even in the face of adversity.

That theoretical base offers no proposals about how it could be taken forward in practice, but it is, in turn, consistent with the practice-based study reported here. Thus, the idea of treating health as a process, and concentrating on the development and use of salutogenic resources and supportive networks in a sociocultural context, appears to be justified in the light of the emerging literature. Furthermore, given the extent of public health concern about widening inequalities in health, social exclusion, rising crime and the costly increase in ill health among numerous vulnerable groups (Benzeval *et al.*, 1995; Lawson, 1997; DoH, 1998), it would seem important for this approach to be encouraged and further developed.

However, the situation in which health visitors work is also influential in determining which approaches they use. At least three factors militate against health visitors implementing this process and context-focused approach within their work. First, in order to allow for the immense variability of individual situations, it privileges lay perceptions of health needs above normatively defined criteria. The testimony of the health visitors was that they had to keep private any interactions in which they afforded priority to the views of their clients above the goals set by their employing authorities. This illustrates both the constraints under which the practitioners operate and the way in which much health visiting work remains hidden.

Second, there is an ever-increasing requirement within the NHS for all professional activities to be counted and accounted for. The mechanisms for this may involve paper records or computerised information systems, but they are all based around the idea of individually focused care (see Cowley, 1994). Activities directed at families, communities or local groups are not recorded; they do not 'count' as clinically focused work so, once more, tend to be hidden and officially discouraged.

The third important factor lies in a circular relationship with the other two, being both their cause and arising from them; it is that health is not regarded as a 'need' within the NHS. One much cited definition suggested that 'need is the ability to benefit from health care' (Stevens and Gabbay, 1991: 20). This provides a starting point for identifying health outcomes; measuring the changes that occur as a result of clinical interventions for people with needs so defined makes it possible to accrue evidence that the health care offered is effective in creating a beneficial change. There is an explicit intention that such evidence of clinical effectiveness should underpin an increasing amount of health service delivery. However, there is a dearth of information about how to evaluate activities directed at creating health or which might target the situation in which an individual lives – their whole family or local area – rather than focusing on individual change. Inevitably, until such a theory base is developed, approaches that can be accounted for most clearly will predominate within a cash-strapped NHS.

Thus, the public health needs arising from the situation of the population served by health visitors and requirements arising from the situation within which these practitioners are employed appear almost diametrically opposed. There is a need for further research to develop the knowledge base on how to assess and measure the effectiveness of interventions across families and communities so that the context and situation can be taken into account. The study reported here offers one small step in that direction.

KEY POINTS

- Grounded theory is a research approach that has proved popular for health visiting studies directed at illuminating processes and the hidden features embedded within health visiting practice. This strategy for handling data in research is recommended when little is known about the field of study; it incorporates the features of theoretical sampling, constant comparative analysis and theoretical saturation.

- There is a dearth of information about how 'health needs' should be specified in relation to health promotion within the well population, in whom no actual change in individual health status is sought. This has implications for assessing needs, planning interventions and measuring outcomes.

44 *The Search for Health Needs*

KEY POINTS (cont'd)

- Treating health as a process fuelled by the accumulation and use of 'resources for health' requires a lifelong, positive-health outlook; interventions are planned for the long term and take account of multiple perspectives.

- Three types of intervention used by health visitors were distinguished by the urgency with which each was required and the length of time the health-enhancing impact of an activity might be expected to last. These were crisis intervention, therapeutic prevention and promoting positive well-being.

- Concentrating on 'crisis interventions' would be counterproductive to the public health as only short-term benefits could be expected. If a caseload is dominated by the need for crisis work, it would be preferable to shift attention to a wider level of health, concentrating on the local community rather than on single individuals with specific needs. This involves focusing on the situation in which families live rather than singling out their problems for attention.

- This way of treating health is internally consistent, supported by various international theories about how health can be created and maintained, and encourages the inclusion of client-led decision-making. However, it is potentially at odds with the short-term, disease-led policies that control NHS spending and service planning.

References

Anderson R. (1984) Health Promotion: An Overview. *European Monographs in Health Education Research* **6**(4): 4–119.

Antonovsky A. (1987) *Unraveling the Mystery of Health: How People Manage Stress and Stay Well.* San Francisco: Jossey Bass.

Antonovsky A. (1993) The structure and properties of the sense of coherence scale. *Social Science and Medicine* **36**(6): 725–33.

Benzeval M., Judge K. and Whitehead M. (1995) *Tackling Inequalities in Health: An Agenda for Action.* London: King's Fund.

Blane D., Brunner E. and Wilkinson R. (1996) *Health and Social Organization.* London: Routledge.

Chalmers K. (1992) Giving and receiving: an empirically derived theory on health visiting practice. *Journal of Advanced Nursing* **17**: 1317–25.

Chalmers K. (1994) Difficult work: health visitors' work with clients in the community. *International Journal of Nursing Studies* **31**: 168–82.

Council for the Education and Training of Health Visitors (CETHV) (1977) *An Investigation into the Principles of Health Visiting.* London: CETHV.

Cowley S. (1991) A symbolic awareness context identified through a grounded theory of health visiting. *Journal of Advanced Nursing* **16**: 648–56.

Cowley S. (1994) Counting practice: the impact of information systems on community nursing. *Journal of Nursing Management* **1**: 273–8.

Cowley S. (1995a) Health-as-process: a health visiting perspective. *Journal of Advanced Nursing* **22**(3): 433–41.

Cowley S. (1995b) In health visiting, the routine visit is one that has passed. *Journal of Advanced Nursing* **22**(2): 276–84.

Cowley S. and Billings J. (1997) *Family Health Needs Project.* London: Department of Nursing Studies, King's College, London.

Cowley S. and Billings J. (1999) Resources revisited: salutogenesis from a lay perspective. *Journal of Advanced Nursing* **29**: 994–1004.

Cuesta C. de la (1993) Fringe work: peripheral work in health visiting. *Sociology of Health and Illness* **15**(5): 667–82.

Cuesta C. de la (1994) Relationships in health visiting: enabling and mediating. *International Journal of Nursing Studies* **31**: 451–9.

Department of Health (DoH) (1989) *Working for Patients.* London: HMSO.

Department of Health (DoH) (1997) *The New NHS: Modern, Dependable.* Cmd 3807. London: Stationery Office.

Department of Health (DoH) (1998) *Our Healthier Nation: A Contract for Health.* Cmd 3852. London: Stationery Office.

Friere P. (1970) *Pedagogy of the Oppressed.* New York: Herder & Herder.

Geissler E. (1984) Crisis: what it is and is not. *Advances in Nursing Science* **7**: 1–9.

Glaser B. (1978) *Theoretical Sensitivity: Advances in the Methodology of Grounded Theory.* Mill Valley, CA: Sociology Press.

Glaser B. and Strauss A. (1967) *The Discovery of Grounded Theory.* Chicago: Aldine.

Guba E. and Lincoln Y. (1985) *Effective Evaluation.* San Francisco, CA: Jossey Bass.

Kolb D. (1984) *Experiential Learning. Experience as a Source of Learning and Development.* Englewood Cliffs, NJ: Prentice Hall.

Lawson R. (1997) *Bills of Health.* Oxford: Radcliffe Medical Press.

Mezirow J. (1981) A critical theory of adult learning and education. *Adult Education* **32**(1): 3–24.

Mustard J.F. (1996) Health and social capital. In Blane D., Brunner E. and Wilkinson R. (eds) *Health and Social Organization.* London: Routledge.

NHS Executive (NHSE) (1996) *Child Health in the Community: A Guide to Good Practice.* London: DoH.

Pearson P. (1991) Clients' perceptions: the use of case studies in developing theory. *Journal of Advanced Nursing* **16**: 521–8.

Putnam R. (1993) *Making Democracy Work: Civic Traditions in Modern Italy.* Princeton, NJ: Princeton University Press.

Rappaport J. (1987) Terms of empowerment/exemplars of prevention: towards a theory for community psychology. *American Journal of Community Psychology* **15**(2): 121–48.

Seedhouse D. (1986) *Health: The Foundations for Achievement.* Chichester: John Wiley & Sons.

Stern P. (1985) Using grounded theory method in nursing research. In Leininger M. (ed.) *Qualitative Research Methods.* Orlando: Grune & Stratton.

Stevens A. and Gabbay J. (1991) Needs assessment needs assessment. *Health Trends* **23**(1): 20–3.

Strauss A. (1987) *Qualitative Analysis for Social Scientists.* Cambridge: Cambridge University Press.

Wilkinson R. (1996) *Unhealthy Societies: The Afflictions of Inequality.* London: Routledge.

World Health Organisation (WHO) (1986) *Ottawa Charter for Health Promotion.* WHO, Geneva.

3

Professional Artistry: The Contribution to the Search for Health Needs

Sheila Twinn

The search for health needs

The search for health needs remains one of the fundamental principles of health visiting practice. The significance of this principle for current and future practice
has been clearly identified both by professional organisations and in government reports and legislation. An
important contribution to the professional literature has
resulted from the work of a group of health visitor educationalists and practitioners set up in 1991 (Twinn and
Cowley, 1992). The group was given the brief to re-examine
the four principles of health visiting practice originally
established in 1974 (CETHV, 1993). The re-examination
was thought necessary as the extensive changes in the
NHS and the subsequent changes in practice had led
practitioners to question whether the principles were still
relevant to client care. The findings of the group reaf-
firmed that the principles remained extremely relevant
to current practice, and this finding has been supported
by more recent professional publications (Campbell *et al.*,
1995). This development coincided with changes in
NHS policy resulting in legislation requiring needs assessment to become part of the service provision of the NHS
(DoH, 1990).

The working group's discussions on the concepts under-pinning the principle of searching for health needs high-lights the complexity of the process. This complexity results in part from the words used to describe the principle. Exten-sive debate was generated among participants by the use of words such as 'search'. 'Search' was considered to imply inquisition, suspicion and aggression rather than partner-ship – the approach to practice currently supported by prac-titioners (Twinn and Cowley, 1992: 16). The term 'need' also generated discussion, particularly concerning the different taxonomies used to inform practice. Despite continued debate, consensus was not achieved in substituting different words for these terms, although agreement was achieved on the significance of the principle to practice.

Billings (1996) argues that the multidimensional nature of needs assessment has contributed to the complexity of the process of searching for health needs. Once again, the definition of the term 'need' provides an example, since sociologists, health economists and epidemiologists each provide a definition of need from their individual perspectives. Campbell *et al.* (1995) provide an example of the multidimensional nature of need by exploring the predictability of need in practice. They suggest that although the starting point for practice may be predicted health needs, as the health visitor works with the family, a multitude of other needs may be uncovered that may have little to do with the previously identified needs.

Cowley *et al.* (1996) broaden the multidimensional nature of assessing need by identifying the significance of context to the definition of need and the process of searching for health needs. They illustrate the importance of context by using the example of a frail elderly person living alone who may have very different needs from a person with a similar health status living with a carer. Research into a range of health topics has demonstrated the effect of context on an individual's or family's health needs. An example is provided by Roberts and Power (1996), who demonstrate that children living in lower socioeconomic families are five times more likely to die from an injury or poisoning than are children in social class I.

The context in which the need occurs also highlights the significance of the political dimension of health visiting practice in searching for health needs. Robinson (1985) argued that this dimension was unique to health visiting in that practitioners had a responsibility actively to search for health needs. At that time, this responsibility raised ethical concerns for some practitioners as needs were identified for which no services were available. However, with the implementation of primary care-led purchasing, health visitors are now in a situation where they have a legitimate role in assessing needs and identifying services to meet those needs, thereby reinforcing the significance of the political dimension of practice, which may come even more to the fore with the proposed introduction of Primary Care Groups (DoH, 1997).

Summers and McKeown (1996) argued that although needs assessment provides health visitors with the opportunity to maximise their skills in public health and health promotion, there is a danger that their role in needs assessment within the GP fundholder primary health care philosophy will isolate them from their traditional public health agenda and previous public health allies. While the implementation of Primary Care Groups under proposed legislation (DoH, 1997) is partly intended to overcome such difficulties, such arguments once more highlight the complexity of the process of searching for health needs.

The final issue for consideration is that of client participation in identifying health needs. Although there is clear acknowledgment that clients should be involved in the process of assessing need, work by authors such as Cowley *et al.* (1996) suggests that clients have been sceptical about the extent to which their views would or could be heard. Consumers also suggested that their view of need was different from that of the professionals. Chalmers (1993), in a study to explore how health visitors search out health needs and promote clients' awareness of health needs, identified four different situations in which these activities occurred. Interestingly, only one of these was client initiated, the other three being professionally led. In addition, this study did not include any clients as subjects, so did

not explore their perception of the process. Evidence such
as this also questions the extent to which clients are truly
involved in identifying health needs.

The evidence does, however, clearly demonstrate not only
the complexity of this principle of health visiting practice,
but also the demands on practitioners to put this principle
into practice effectively. Indeed, this involves skills such as
those identified in the study by Chalmers (1993) as well as
extensive levels of knowledge from which to make the skilled
professional judgements required of practitioners frequently
working in situations that may be unpredictable, ambiguous
or anomalous (Cowley, 1995). The uncertainty and uniqueness of these client–health visitor interventions highlight
the significance of the level of competence of the practitioner in managing the situation effectively.

Competence in professional practice

Fish and Twinn (1997) suggest that confusion exists within
professional education in the understanding of competence in professional practice. The authors use the definition provided by Carr (1997) to describe competence as
working 'in a broadly principled, reflective and informed
way', rather than in terms of prespecifiable, discrete
itemised skills or competences. Indeed, it is the interpretation of competence in terms of a skills-based approach
resulting in the implementation of a routinised approach
to practice that has created criticism of professional practice and practitioners (Schön, 1992). The definition of
competence in practice thus requires practitioners to have
not only the professional and personal knowledge from
which to develop a principled approach to practice, but
also the intuition and creativity required of practitioners
to make professional judgements that respond to the
uniqueness of the clinical situation.

This definition of competence highlights the significance of the concept of professional artistry to competence in practice (Schön, 1987). Drawing from the work
of Schön, professional artistry is defined as the intuitive

knowing-in-practice by which practitioners make sense of the practice setting to inform professional judgements from which strategies and practice are determined. Intuitive knowing-in-practice refers to the synthesis of the practitioner's understanding of practice phenomena (complexity, uncertainty, instability, uniqueness and value conflict) in guiding the outcome of professional decision-making and is therefore essential to competence in practice (Twinn, 1991).

In the author's view, professional artistry is particularly relevant to the processes involved in searching for health needs since it enables practitioners to use their intuitive knowing-in-practice to make sense of the practice setting and to make professional judgements to inform strategies in practice. The processes used by practitioners to inform their professional judgements make a major contribution to their level of professional competence. The extent to which practitioners achieve the required level of competence in making professional judgements plays an important role in the quality of health visiting practice. An interest in these issues led the author to carry out a study to investigate the understanding of competence in health visiting practice and the assessment of competence in student health visitors (Twinn, 1989). The study is detailed below; the suspected importance of professional artistry to competence, especially in relation to the search for health needs, will be highlighted as the results and implications are discussed.

The research study

The aim of this study was thus to address an important issue affecting the quality of health visiting practice: to examine the relationship between the interpretation of professional practice and the process of assessing competence in practice in student health visitors. To achieve this aim, the following objectives were identified:

- to analyse the different paradigms of health visiting practice currently used by practitioners;
- to identify and analyse the current methods and procedures used to assess students' competence in practice;
- to identify and analyse the interaction and relationship between the processes and individuals involved in the assessment process;
- to identify and analyse the learning needs of the individuals involved in carrying out the assessment process;
- to develop a theoretical framework for the process of assessing competence in practice.

In order to achieve these objectives, a multistage mixed research design was used. As illustrated in Figure 3.1, the research design consisted of an initial survey of all colleges offering a health visitor course in England and a case study. The discussion in this chapter will focus on the case study component of the research design since the findings from this part of the study are particularly relevant to the contribution of professional artistry to the search for health needs.

Although a case study approach was selected partly because of the lack of previous research within the topic area, the main reason for its selection was that it allowed an in-depth analysis of the research question in one particular setting. Indeed, Yin (1994) argues that case study designs are particularly relevant when there has been little research in the context of the real-life setting and the boundaries between the phenomena being investigated are not clearly evident. One of the criticisms of the case study design is that findings cannot be generalised to other settings. However, Yin (1994) argues that the theory developed from the findings of a case study can be generalised to other settings and used to predict outcomes and behaviours.

Another important issue to consider in case study design is the unit of analysis. Yin (1989) defines the units of analysis as the significant subunits within the case study. Within this case study, it was important to include all those involved in the process of assessing the student's competence to practise. This process involved the community practice teacher (CPT), responsible for the student's education and training

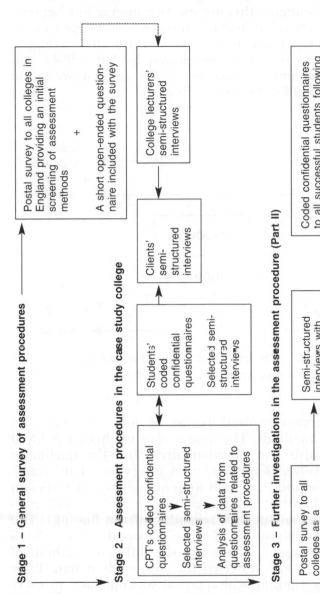

Stage 1 – General survey of assessment procedures

Postal survey to all colleges in England providing an initial screening of assessment methods

+

A short open-ended questionnaire included with the survey

Stage 2 – Assessment procedures in the case study college

College lecturers' semi-structured interviews

Clients' semi-structured interviews

Students' coded confidential questionnaires

Selected semi-structured interviews

CPTs coded confidential questionnaires

Selected semi-structured interviews

Analysis of data from questionnaires related to assessment procedures

Stage 3 – Further investigations in the assessment procedure (Part II)

Coded confidential questionnaires to all successful students following completion of the course

Semi-structured interviews with CPTs and students

Postal survey to all colleges as a screening procedure

Figure 3.1   The stages of the research design

in the clinical setting, college lecturers, clients and, of course, the students themselves. The interaction between these four sets of individuals involved in the process of assessing competence to practise is illustrated in Figure 3.2. Using the definition developed by Yin (1994), this provided four units of analysis for the study, resulting in a single embedded case study design.

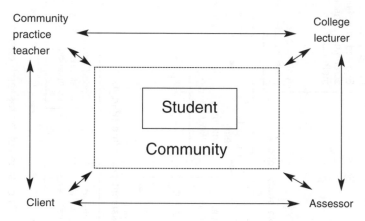

Figure 3.2   The interaction of the individuals involved in the assessment of practical competence

Data collection involved the use of both qualitative and quantitative methods. The quantitative methods employed student records and questionnaires, and the qualitative methods involved semi-structured interviews. The combination of methods was used to generate data of sufficient depth to achieve the objectives for the study as well as to maximise the validity and reliability of the findings. The issues of reliability and validity are discussed in more detail later in the chapter. The use of the different methods of data collection also reflected the case study design. Prior to data collection, ethical approval was obtained to carry out the study, and written informed consent was obtained from all participants in the study.

Quantitative methods of data collection

The quantitative methods of data collection involved the use of a confidential questionnaire and student records. The questionnaire was an important initial stage of the case study design and was administered to both CPTs and students. A confidential coded questionnaire was circulated by post to the sample of CPTs and students. The questionnaire for the CPTs consisted of two parts. The first part involved a professional biography, including information about the teacher's practice, and the second part asked questions on the assessment procedure. The questionnaire involved both open-ended and closed questions.

The coded confidential questionnaire circulated to the students consisted of three parts. The first part included demographic details, the second part questions on the students' experience in fieldwork practice and the third part questions on the assessment of their competence in practice. Once again, both open-ended and closed questions were used. The questionnaires were coded to allow the selection of a sample of both students and CPTs to participate in a semi structured interview. Both questionnaires were piloted with a group of students and CPTs from another training institution prior to their administration. No amendments were required following the pilot study.

The second quantitative method of data collection employed was the student assessment procedure completed by the CPT to assess the student's competence in practice. This was used to supplement the data obtained from the questionnaires and semi-structured interviews.

Qualitative methods of data collection

Semi-structured interviews were used as the method of qualitative data collection and were undertaken with a sample of CPTs, students, clients and college lecturers. For those interviews undertaken with the CPTs and students, the interview guide was developed from the analysis of the questionnaire data as well as from a review of the literature. These sources also contributed to the interview guides developed for the client and lecturer samples. All the interviews were tape-recorded and lasted approximately 45 minutes. For all four samples, a pilot interview was undertaken prior to the main study to ensure a correct interview technique and the appropriate sequencing of the topics in the interview.

Sampling in the case study

The sampling methods in the case study reflected the methods of data collection and therefore varied with the different stages of the case study. A total sample was used for the administration of the questionnaire. This involved a sample of 27 CPTs and 27 students. Purposive sampling was used to select the sample of CPTs and students for the semi-structured interview. Following the analysis of the data from the questionnaire completed by the CPTs, 13 were selected for interview. The criteria for selection were identified from the findings in the questionnaire to ensure the selection of informants who could contribute to the depth of data required from the interviews. Indeed, Morse (1991) argues that an appropriate selection of informants is essential in ensuring the quality of data in qualitative research. The student sample selected for interview was determined by the CPT sample so that the student's perception of the process could be matched to that of the CPT. This was important as, in health visiting education, one CPT generally takes the responsibility for one student's fieldwork experience, developing a close working relationship with that student.

For the lecturer sample, a total population was once more used as the health visiting lecturing staff in the college consisted of five members. Although a small number, this was considered appropriate to supplement the data obtained from the postal survey in the first stage of the study, particularly since debate over the adequacy of the sample size for qualitative studies continues (Sandelowski, 1995). The final stage of the case study involved semi-structured interviews with a sample of clients. An oppor-

tunistic sampling method was used by requesting 11
selected CPTs each to choose three clients who had been
involved with the student's learning experience during
fieldwork practice. This provided a sample of 33 clients
who agreed to participate in the semi-structured interview.
Although there are some criticisms of using this sampling
method (Morse, 1991), it was considered the most appropriate for this group in the case study, particularly as the
CPTs were selected for their perceived competence in
health visiting practice and teaching ability.

Validity and reliability of the research design

One of the great strengths of using case study design has
also been described as a potential weakness. The opportunity for the researcher to gain an in-depth knowledge of
the thoughts, feelings and actions of individuals in a specific
situation may create such familiarity with the phenomenon
under question that objectivity may become particularly
difficult for the researcher (Polit and Hungler, 1995). In
order to address such issues and enhance validity and reliability methods, triangulation was used in the study (Kimchi
et al., 1991).

Polit and Hungler (1995: 655) describe triangulation as
'the use of multiple methods or perspectives to collect and
interpret data about some phenomenon, to converge on
an accurate representation of reality'. Four major types of
triangulation are commonly used: data, investigator, theory
and methods. Methods triangulation was used in this study
as a method of confirming the accuracy of the data sets
obtained from the study and involved the use of questionnaires, semi-structured interviews and the students'
practice reports. Convergence of these data was undertaken to add to the depth and breadth of the understanding
of the findings generated from the study (Knafl and Breitmayer, 1991).

The reliability of the data was enhanced by tape-recording
all the interviews and by only one researcher being involved
in the transcription and analysis of the interview data. In

addition, the use of a semi-structured interview enhanced the consistency of the data collected from the informants. Although the questionnaire was prepiloted to test for the validity of the questions, it was not tested for reliability, and this had to be taken into account when interpreting the results. The use of coded questionnaires, however, provided the opportunity for checking both the validity and reliability of the data with the data obtained from the semi-structured interviews.

An analysis was undertaken of both the qualitative and quantitative data. Because of the nature of the question-naire, descriptive statistics were used to measure frequencies and means. Content analysis of the qualitative data was undertaken using the process suggested by Polit and Hungler (1995). The findings from the qualitative data have generally been used to explore the implications of the interpretation of practice on the process of the search for health needs, in particular the contribution of professional artistry. The implications have been considered from two different perspectives, reflecting the units of analysis in the case study design. The findings therefore focus on the clients' and health visitors' perspective of the interpretation of practice and the implications of these findings for the search for health needs.

The clients' interpretation of practice

From the opportunistic sample of 33 clients, 24 agreed to participate in the semi-structured interviews. Despite an opportunistic sampling, the informants represented a range of social class, three of the sample being unemployed. All the informants were women and all had young children, reflecting a traditional interpretation of health visiting practice. Two of the sample were single parents, and only two came from an ethnic minority background. At the request of the women, all the interviews were conducted in their home since they said they felt more relaxed and at ease in their own surroundings. All agreed to the interviews being tape-recorded, and although one woman described the tape-recorder as 'putting you off slightly', no one expressed any anxiety, either overtly or covertly, about the tape-recording of the interviews.

Within the current framework of health visiting, a client's interpretation of professional practice generally results from direct contact with an individual practitioner (Kelly, 1996). Since earlier research had demonstrated the difficulties experienced by some clients in describing the role of the health visitor (Clark, 1984; Watson, 1986), the participants were asked to describe any aspects of health visiting that they had found either particularly helpful or unhelpful. From these experiences, it was clear that these women were able to construct their own interpretation of health visiting practice. In the analysis of these experiences, four particular practice categories were identified: advising, providing information, offering support and client advocacy. In order to illustrate the implications of the interpretation of practice for the search for health needs, the practice categories of advising and offering support have been selected.

The category of advice-giving was identified from examples of both helpful and unhelpful experiences. It is perhaps significant to the search for health needs that the majority of findings on advice-giving were obtained from the negative experiences of the women. Negative experiences particularly related to conflicting or inappropriate advice. Frequently, conflicting advice was given about infant feeding, and this was highlighted as a source of distress and anger by several women. One described her feelings saying:

> having my own ideas and sometimes I sit in here and think yes but I'm not going to do that. (Client 20: 102)

Another said:

> if their advice had been contrary to what I believed I wouldn't take it... you have to draw the line with health visitors. (Client 11: 84).

Where positive experiences of advice-giving were cited, they generally related to specific health problems such as sleep difficulties. Clients describing these experiences could be divided into two categories. The first consisted of those who wanted to be told what to do, and the second of those who wanted to know the advice but would then make their own decision about managing the situation. The need for the advice to be down to earth and practical was clearly identified. Both the positive and the negative experiences highlight the need for practitioners to draw on their intuitive knowing-in-practice so that they can make sense of the individual practice situation to inform professional judgements and guide the strategies used in practice.

Offering support emerged from the data analysis as a particularly important role of the health visitor. Support was described as listening, acting as a 'sounding board' and responding to the expressed needs of the client. Clients described acting as a sounding board within the context of enabling decisions about issues such as immunisation and solving personal problems. Others described the importance of the practitioner responding to expressed need, with one client saying:

> she came when I screamed for her... or I don't think Lisa would have lived six months. (Client 13: 120)

Another illustrated this finding by commenting:

> asking someone to come visit – no matter how trivial she's not going to think you're making a fuss about nothing. (Client 10: 28)

Indeed, the importance and value attached to the role of listener was demonstrated throughout the data, highlighting the significance of the support role in the client's interpretation of practice. It is perhaps interesting that research indicates that practitioners find effective listening difficult (Sefi, 1985; May, 1990; Kendall, 1993). This finding has significant implications for the search for health needs.

From the data obtained from the topic of child protection, providing support also emerged as an important role for the health visitor. Clients were asked whether they saw the health visitor as having responsibility for monitoring the care that parents provided for their children. Interestingly, although only three of the women felt that they were being monitored, a spontaneous response from the majority of the women was that although they did not feel that their care was being monitored, they had friends and relatives who did. The extent to which these women were projecting their feelings onto a third person must be considered. It is important to note, however, that one woman described her feelings thus:

> No I've never felt that but I'm sure they do – I think it's a credit to them that I don't feel as if they are doing it. (Client 4: 200)

Once again, this example highlights the significance of the professional competence of the health visitors in effectively searching for health needs. Importantly, in addition, both these practice categories highlight the significance of the personal attributes of the health visitor to the process of searching for health needs.

The negative experiences identified in the practice categories in the data illustrate the importance of the personal attributes of the health visitor. When clients were asked to identify the attributes of an effective practitioner, the most frequently cited attribute was that she or he should be easy to talk to. The second two items, each cited seven times, were a friendly manner and being a good listener. Interestingly, 50 per cent of the sample identified attributes that directly influence the quality of the client–practitioner relationship, which has implications for the effectiveness of the health visitor in searching for health needs. Indeed, one woman summed up the importance of the personal attributes of the health visitor as follows:

> [they should] like children, like people, quite patient because all mums ask silly questions and don't need to be snapped at in reply... likes babies generally friendly – quite outgoing and extrovert without being nosey – they've got to have their heads screwed on... know what they're watching out for. (Client 4: 58)

It is also important to observe that although women described the importance of liking the health visitor, she may have nothing to offer as a health visitor. Evidence such as this highlights not only the complex issues involved in the client–health visitor relationship, but also that clients recognise and can articulate competence in practice.

The argument presented by Schön (1987) suggests that it is the process employed by practitioners in their understanding of knowing-in-action, tacit knowing and intuition when making professional judgements that partly distinguishes competent from incompetent practice. The findings of this study indicate that the process is also influenced by the attitudes and personal attributes of the health visitor, which implicitly influence the practitioner's use of intuition. Indeed, the data highlight the significance of the intuitive knowing-in-practice as well as the personal attributes and attitudes of the health visitor for the outcome of practice strategies, particularly within the context of searching for health needs.

Health visitors' interpretation of practice

In order to reflect the design of the case study, the health visitors' interpretation of professional practice draws on data obtained from both CPTs and students. The data were obtained from the confidential questionnaires administered to the CPTs and the semi-structured interviews. From the total population of 27 CPTs, 24 completed the questionnaire, a response rate of 89 per cent. All 13 CPTs selected for the interview agreed to participate. The data for the students were obtained from the questionnaire and semi-structured interviews. From the total population of students, 26 completed the confidential questionnaire, a response rate of 96 per cent. Twelve out of the 13 students agreed to participate in the semi-structured interview. The findings from the data from the CPTs and students have been presented independently so that a comparison of the interpretation of practice can be made.

It had been anticipated by the researcher that one particular question asking the CPTs' opinion of the most important health visiting skills would provide the data from which the CPTs' interpretation of practice could be identified. Unfortunately, this question had been interpreted in different ways by the CPT sample, thus making the data invalid for analysis. It is interesting that this phenomenon had not been identified in either the prepiloting or piloting of the questionnaire. In order to analyse the interpretation of practice, it was therefore necessary to sift through the data obtained from other questions on the questionnaire and the interview data to categorise those areas of practice consistently identified by the CPTs.

From the interview data, those health visiting skills identified by more than one informant included home visiting, the formation of relationships, communication and record-keeping. It is interesting that record-keeping, a very specific skill, was identified among the practice categories. This finding may reflect the increasing emphasis placed on child protection issues at the time of the data collection, in particular identifying and preventing child abuse. These data suggest that child protection issues may provide an important focus for the interpretation of practice. It is important to note that the skill of assessment – of families, individuals or need – was not explicitly identified by the CPTs.

The data from the questionnaire, however, presented a rather different picture. One question specifically asked the CPTs to identify criteria other than health visiting skills that they used to assess the practical competence of students. The analysis of the data identified practice categories reflecting the wider issues of professional knowledge and including attributes such as tact, discretion, sensitivity and the students' perception of the needs of clients. Findings such as these raise interesting questions concerning the role of assessment and the search for health needs in the interpretation of practice, particularly as research suggests that the assessment of a family's vulnerability is an essential component of health visiting practice (Appleton, 1995).

It is important to observe that these practice issues were also cited by the CPTs as the most difficult areas in which to assess the students' competence in practice. The four specific categories identified by the CPTs included self-awareness, perception, sensitivity and the ability to, relate to clients. These categories clearly contribute to the students' ability to develop the concept of professional artistry. The significance of the student's personality, particularly his or her ability to develop an effective relationship with clients, emerged as an important finding from the interview data. Indeed, all but one of the 13 informants acknowledged that personality influenced the competence of the practitioner. This finding suggests that elements making up professional artistry implicitly play a role in the interpretation of practice.

It is, however, significant that the CPTs expressed greater concern about the students' level of knowledge in the very specific areas of health visiting practice rather than the students' potential to develop the concept of professional artistry. Evidence such as this perhaps supports the argument put forward by Schön (1987: 13) that terms such as 'intuition' 'serve not to open up inquiry but to close it off'. The findings also suggest that the CPTs experienced a degree of conflict in their interpretation of practice. The explicit interpretation focuses on a skills-based approach to practice, whereas implicitly the significance of the components contributing to professional artistry was also considered to be essential to the interpretation of competence in practice. Findings such as these are important to the interpretation of practice and in searching for health needs, particularly when the client's interpretation of practice is considered.

The students were also not asked a specific question, either in the questionnaire or the semi-structured interview, relating directly to their interpretation of practice. Once again, it was necessary to sift through the data to identify specific practice issues to demonstrate their individual interpretations. One question in the questionnaire, asking students to identify the criteria that should be used to assess their competence in practice, identified practice issues considered to be significant to the students' interpretation of practice. Those criteria identified by more than one respondent were client satisfaction, a realistic prioritising of client's needs, communication and personal relationships. Indeed, one student described health visiting as 'all to do with relationships and how you interact with people'.

The concept of client need and a client-centred approach to practice was picked up as an issue for discussion in the semi-structured interviews. The frustration experienced by students when their perception of client need differed from that of the CPT was identified. This was illustrated by a student describing her feelings when she considered that a particular client was exhibiting signs of depression, which was disputed by her CPT. This illustration not only demonstrates the different interpretation of practitioners, in particular in searching for health needs, but also the significance of these processes to the quality of health visiting practice.

Important practice issues could also be identified from the data obtained from the discussion with the students on areas of fieldwork practice they found particularly difficult. One issue was that of giving advice to parents about the many different topics related to child health. Other issues, however, could be categorised within the broader definition of professional knowledge and included forming relationships, knocking on unknown doors not knowing what was on the other side, listening and planning priorities. Once again, these practice issues have implications for the interpretation of practice. Indeed, although the findings were obtained from questions not directly related to practice, there are clear indications of the students' interpretation of practice, and although there were commonalities between the students' interpretation and that of the CPTs', differences were also identified.

These differences may in part be accounted for by the fact that neither group were directly asked to describe their interpretation of practice, and the sifting of data to answer this question may have contributed to a different focus within the data of each group. It is, however, significant that both groups identified the practice issues of client need and the client–health visitor relationship in their interpretation of practice. Client need, although obviously fundamental to the search for health needs, must be considered from the client's perspective. The competence required to form effective relationships draws heavily on personal characteristics such as sensitivity, self-awareness and perception, which are prerequisites for the development of professional artistry. Interestingly, these particular practice issues appear to reflect those valued by the client sample in this study, demonstrating the importance of these practice issues to high-quality health visiting practice. The findings therefore suggest that professional artistry has a major contribution to make to the implementation of the principle of searching for health needs. The literature, however, indicates that scepticism remains about the true contribution of professional artistry to the search for health needs. The final section of this chapter will, therefore, attempt to consider the recommendations for practice to facilitate the development and recognition of the art of searching for health needs and the contribution of this process to the outcome of practice.

The art of identifying health needs: implications for practice

The findings from this study indicate a degree of conflict in practitioners' interpretation of practice. The conflict appears, in part, to be a response to the significance attached to the belief that concepts of health visiting can be operationalised, measured, quantified and therefore made scientific, thereby contributing to the development of a professional discipline of practice. Practitioners, however, also clearly identified the significance of personal attributes and characteristics in professional knowledge, demonstrating a belief that the concepts are unique and particular to each individual situation and therefore implicitly associated with the artistry of practice. The definition of competence in practice given earlier in the chapter, stating that practitioners work 'in a broadly principled, reflective and informed way' (adapted from Carr by Fish and Twinn, 1997: 49), highlights the significance of artistry to the process of searching for health needs. This is particularly so since this process requires practitioners to make sense of a range of practice criteria to inform their professional judgements. This interpretation of competence identifies three important implications for health visiting practice:

- the acknowledgment of the essential role of professional artistry in searching for health needs;
- the fundamental role of education in developing the concept of professional artistry;
- the need for research to articulate the contribution of professional artistry to searching for health needs.

The essential role of professional artistry in searching for health needs

In the author's view, the data indicate that some of the problems in searching for health needs have arisen from practitioners attempting to legitimise the professional status of health visiting by focusing practice on a set of competences considered to be appropriate to practice. This has led to practitioners negating the art of practice and adopting routinised and mechanistic approaches to practice. This approach to practice fails to allow practitioners to identify needs from the clients' perspective since it fails to acknowledge the significance of practice criteria in informing professional judgements. Importantly, this approach also fails to allow health visitors to adapt their practice to the changing needs of the context in which they are working or appraise their own performance in practice.

It is failures such as these that influence the effectiveness of searching for health needs. Indeed, to achieve a successful outcome for practice, it is essential that practitioners move away from instrumental problem-solving in which practitioners attempt to fit practice situations into professional knowledge by either ignoring issues that do not correspond to defined categories or forcing the situation to fit available techniques. A conceptual framework for health visiting practice that acknowledges the essential role of professional artistry is one way of effectively searching for health needs (Twinn, 1996). This approach to a conceptual framework for practice, however, requires the recognition of intuitive knowledge as a legitimate element of professional practice and has implications for both education and research in health visiting.

The fundamental role of education in developing the concept of professional artistry

Although there is little doubt surrounding the important role that education plays in preparing students to search for health needs, the findings from this study once again demonstrate a degree of conflict for practitioners. The data generally demonstrate the emphasis placed on the skills and professional knowledge required for practice. However, practitioners, although repeatedly acknowledging the significance of interpersonal skills, self-awareness and intuitive knowledge for professional judgements, did not consider these characteristics to be legitimate criteria for questioning the students' competence in practice and therefore failing a student. Evidence such as this highlights the need for education to give equal emphasis to the values and beliefs underpinning practice if students are to develop the ability to respond effectively to complex and changing practice environments. In this approach to education, the role of the CPT is particularly important in coaching the students through a range of practice situations.

Fish and Twinn (1997) describe a framework developed to help CPTs to manage the complexities of this process during the debriefing discussions in student supervision. The framework, referred to as the strands of reflection, facilitates CPTs' exploration of the values and beliefs underpinning a range of practice situations with students. The need for a change in focus in education and the interpretation of practice highlights the importance of practitioners articulating the contribution of professional artistry to the outcome of practice and the search for health needs in particular.

The need to articulate the contribution of professional artistry to the search for health needs

Professional artistry, although essential to competence in practice, is one of the most complex elements of professional practice. The characteristics of professional artistry are perhaps some of the most difficult to distinguish and evaluate through clinical research. However, the need to investigate the contribution of professional artistry to the process of searching for health needs highlights the demand for research in this area.

Schön (1987) suggests that professional artistry is implicitly linked with reflection-in-action, which requires practitioners continually to analyse previous practice experience and, from these experiences, to formulate hypotheses that can be tested by experimental action in practice. This experimental action in practice allows practitioners to test out the different processes and activities involved in the process in making informed professional judgements. The setting of hypotheses in the practice setting also highlights the importance of problem-setting rather than problem-solving to the development of clinical practice. Although a complex research process, in the author's view, developing research activities within the context of reflection-in-action enables practitioners to articulate the processes involved in effectively searching for health needs. It would also assist in the evaluation of the contribution of professional artistry to the outcome of the search for health needs and, implicitly, the quality of health visiting practice.

Conclusion

In the author's view, the implications for practice highlight some important issues for consideration by practitioners in the search for health needs. This is particularly so as the nature of health visiting practice becomes increasingly diverse and the processes involved in searching for health needs become more complex. These issues include the interpretation of competence in practice and the fundamental role of professional education in determining that interpretation of competence, as well as the significance of research in articulating and developing the processes involved in the implementation of that interpretation of practice. Indeed, it appears that research plays an essential role not only in allowing practitioners to determine the contribution of professional artistry to the search for health needs, but also in the implications of this interpretation of practice for the quality of client care.

KEY POINTS

- The concept of professional artistry is an essential component of the search for health needs if that process is to meet clients' health needs.

- The concept of professional artistry is fundamental to the interpretation of competence in practice if high-quality care is to be achieved in identifying and meeting clients' health needs.

- The need to undertake further research to determine the contribution of professional artistry to practice, in particular to the search for health needs, is essential to the development of high-quality practice.

- The need to use a research methodology, such as the case study design, that acknowledges the complexities of investigating phenomena within the real-life setting is highlighted. Implicit within this design is the contribution of multiple methods of data collection to informing the outcome of the study.

References

Appleton J. (1995) Health visitor assessment of vulnerability. *Health Visitor* **68**(6): 228–31.

Billings J. (1996) Assessing health needs. In Twinn S., Roberts B. and Andrews S. (eds) *Community Health Care Nursing.* Oxford: Butterworth Heinemann.

Campbell F., Cowley S. and Buttigieg M. (1995) *Weights and Measures: Outcomes and Evaluation in Health Visiting.* London: HVA.

Carr D. (1997) Cited in Fish D. and Twinn S. *Quality Clinical Supervision in the Health Care Professions.* Oxford: Butterworth Heinemann, p. 49.

Chalmers K. (1993) Searching for health needs: the work of health visiting. *Journal of Advanced Nursing* **18**: 900–11.

Clark J. (1984) Mothers' perceptions of health visitors. *Health Visitor* **57**(9): 265–8.

Council for the Education and Training of Health Visitors (CETHV) (1993) *An Investigation into the Principles of Health Visiting.* London: ENB.

Cowley S. (1995) In health visiting, a routine visit is one that has passed. *Journal of Advanced Nursing* **22**: 276–84.

Cowley S., Bergen A., Young K. and Kavanagh A. (1996) Establishing a framework for research: the example of needs assessment. *Journal of Clinical Nursing* **5**: 53–61.

Department of Health (DoH) (1990) *The NHS and Community Care Act.* London: HMSO.

Department of Health (DoH) (1997) *The New NHS: Modern, Dependable.* London: Stationery Office.

Fish D. and Twinn S. (1997) *Quality Clinical Supervision in the Health Care Professions.* Oxford: Butterworth Heinemann.

Kelly C. (1996) Public perceptions of a health visitor. *International Journal of Nursing Studies* **33**(3): 285–96.

Kendall S. (1993) How do health visitors provide advice? *Journal of Clinical Nursing* **2**(2): 103–9.

Kimchi J., Polivka B. and Sabol Stevenson J. (1991) Triangulation: operational definitions. *Nursing Research* (Nov/Dec): 364–6.

Knafl K. and Breitmayer B. (1991) Triangulation in qualitative research: issues in conceptual clarity and purpose. In Morse J. (ed.) *Qualitative Nursing Research: A Contemporary Dialogue.* Newbury Park, CA: Sage.

May C. (1990) Research on nurse–patient relationships: problems of theory, problems of theory. *Journal of Advanced Nursing* **15**: 307–15.

Morse J. (1991) Strategies in sampling. In Morse J. (ed.) *Qualitative Nursing Research: A Contemporary Dialogue.* Newbury Park, CA: Sage.

Polit D. and Hungler B. (1995) *Nursing Research: Principles and Methods,* (5th edn). Philadelphia, PA: J.B. Lippincott.

Roberts I. and Power C. (1996) Does the decline in child injury mortality vary by social class? A comparison of class specific mortality in 1981 and 1991. *British Medical Journal* **313**: 784–6.

Robinson J. (1985) Health visiting and health. In White R. (ed.) *Political Issues in Nursing,* Vol. 1. Chichester: John Wiley & Sons.

Sandelowski M. (1995) Focus on qualitative methods: sample size in qualitative research. *Research in Nursing and Health* **18**: 179–83.

Schön D. (1987) *Educating the Reflective Practitioner.* San Francisco, CA: Jossey-Bass.

Schön D. (1992) The crisis of professional knowledge and the pursuit of an epistemology of practice. *Journal of Interprofessional Care* 6(1): 49–63.

Sefi S. (1985) The First Visit: A Study of Health Visitor/Mother Verbal Interaction. Unpublished MA dissertation, University of Warwick.

Summers A. and McKeown K. (1996) Health needs assessment in primary care: a role for health visitors. *Health Visitor* 69(8): 323–4.

Twinn S. (1989) Change and Conflict in Health Visiting Practice: Dilemmas in Assessing the Professional Competence of Student Health Visitors. Unpublished PhD thesis, Institute of Education University of London.

Twinn S. (1991) Conflicting paradigms of health visiting: a continuing debate for professional practice. *Journal of Advanced Nursing* 16: 966–73.

Twinn S. (1996) Philosophies, structures and traditions: implications for a framework for practice. In Twinn S., Roberts B. and Andrews S. (eds) *Community Health Care Nursing*. Oxford: Butterworth Heinemann.

Twinn S. and Cowley S. (eds) (1992) *The Principles of Health Visiting: A Re-examination*. London: HVA/UKSC.

Watson E. (1986) A mismatch of goals? *Health Visitor* 59(3): 75–7.

Yin R.K. (1989) *Case Study Research. Design and Method* (rev. edn). Newbury Park, CA: Sage.

Yin R.K. (1994) *Case Study Research. Design and Method* (2nd edn). Newbury Park, CA: Sage.

4

Using Guidelines to Prioritise Families who Need Additional Health Visiting Support

Jane V. Appleton

This chapter will explore the use of guidelines in health visiting practice in the 'search for health needs'. Its main focus is the practice guidelines that are issued to health visitors to assist in the identification of vulnerable families, with the intention of identifying 'health need' and increasing health visiting intervention and support to families. The chapter will initially examine the current NHS focus on 'evidence-based practice' and the increasing moves towards clinical practice guideline development among health professionals, particularly those in the health visiting service. The key policy initiatives that have influenced this move will be highlighted.

A national study will then be described that has attempted to evaluate the clinical practice guidelines issued to health visitors to assist in the identification of families requiring increased health visitor support and intervention. In a needs-led service, this is an essential step towards establishing whether current clinical practice guidelines are valid and potentially helpful to practitioners. This chapter offers one approach for analysing clinical practice guidelines and describes the strengths and weaknesses of the critique and analysis tool developed for the study.

The most important findings that have emerged from the research will then be examined in the context of contemporary community nursing practice. Finally, key pointers for health visiting practice will be identified.

Clinical practice guidelines

Over the past decade, there has been considerable interest in the development and use of clinical practice guidelines in medicine and nursing. However, confusion over terminology often exists in the fact that the terms 'protocol', 'clinical practice guideline', 'local guideline' and 'health care/nursing standards' are often used interchangeably in community nursing practice. It is perhaps useful to clarify the meaning of these terms. Protocols and standards differ from clinical guidelines in that they are formal written procedures addressing the management of patient/ client care in specific situations. Standards are written in the form of 'an authoritative statement' (Sullivan and Mann, 1994: 413), which should include an objective of care and detailed guidance on how to reach that objective (Duff *et al.*, 1996).

Clinical guidelines are, however, 'systematically developed statements to assist practitioner and patient decisions about appropriate health care for specific clinical circumstances' (Field and Lohr, 1992: 2). Grimshaw and Russell (1993) and Antrobus and Brown (1996) recommend the need for clinical guidelines to be developed from sound research evidence combined with expert opinion. Eddy (1990) has provided a useful distinction between standards and guidelines, stating that standards describe appropriate health care and should be adhered to in all circumstances, whereas clinical guidelines, while providing guidance to the practitioner, allow flexibility and acknowledge professional discretion (Grimshaw and Russell, 1993). It is perhaps important to clarify that clinical practice guidelines should not be viewed as a replacement for professional judgement but that their purpose is to aid the decision-making processes (Sullivan and Mann, 1994; Carruthers, 1995). Where clinical practice guidelines are adapted for use by individual Trusts, these are known as local guidelines and often contain more detailed operational specifications (Grimshaw and Russell, 1993; RCN, 1995).

In the UK NHS, there is an increasing move towards developing clinical guidelines to improve standards of patient and client care (University of Leeds, 1994; Deighan and Hitch, 1995). The current focus on 'evidence-based medicine' and more recently 'evidence-based health care' has recommended the need to develop clinical practice guidelines based on evidence from randomised controlled research designs (Russell and Grimshaw, 1995; Sackett and Rosenberg, 1995). Evidence-based practice (Sakett *et al.*, 1996: 71) is defined as:

> the conscientious, explicit and judicious use of current best evidence in making decisions about the care of individual patients. The practice of evidence-based health care means integrating individual clinical expertise with the best available external, clinical evidence from systematic research.

The overall purpose of evidence-based clinical guidelines is to ensure that clinical practice is guided and underpinned by sound research evidence (Von Degenberg, 1996) and scientifically valid criteria.

Within nursing, much emphasis has traditionally been placed on the development of practice standards, yet since the mid-1990s there has been considerable interest in the potential of clinical practice guidelines. A consequence is that clinical guidelines are being introduced into many areas of nursing practice, for example pressure sore prevention and the management and treatment of leg ulcers. These clinical practice guidelines clearly have potential for providing guidance for patient/client assessment and searching for health needs. However, what is particularly significant is the fact that very few research studies have been undertaken to evaluate the effectiveness of the clinical practice guidelines currently in use in nursing practice (RCN, 1995).

A growth in the development of clinical guidelines has been further stimulated by moves from the NHS Executive (NHSE) to recommend that guidelines should be used to inform contracts (NHSME, 1993; NHSE, 1994). More recently, Antrobus and Brown (1996: 39) have again brought this issue into the spotlight by stating that 'rather than focusing purchasing procedures on levels of activity, health care commissioners should explore the possibility of purchasing guidelines and protocols'. Some researchers have also outlined the possibility that clinical practice guidelines could reduce variations in clinical practices as well as promoting more cost-effective care (Carruthers, 1995; Klazinga, 1995; Russell and Grimshaw, 1995). However, Hutchinson *et al.* (1995: 50) have been more cautious by highlighting that, in fact:

> many clinical guidelines do not show an explicit link between the evidence on which they are based and the recommendations contained in the guidelines, [and second] there are relatively few examples... where guidelines have been shown to have a demonstrable and sustained positive effect on health care.

Anecdotal evidence suggests that a problem with many clinical guidelines being used in hospital and community nursing practice is the fact that many are formed without sufficient empirical data, focusing instead on so-called 'expert opinion' (Russell and Grimshaw, 1995: 78). Thus, where clinical practice guidelines currently exist in nursing, the need to evaluate their quality seems a particularly pertinent issue, especially in view of current research and policy initiatives stressing the potential of clinical guidelines for promoting clinical effectiveness and high-quality client care.

Current issues in health visiting

Despite the current emphasis on community health care services, official figures indicate that the number of practising health visitors is in decline (HVA, 1994), and the 1998 Community Practitioners' and Health Visitors' Association Workforce survey indicated that nearly a quarter of health visitors are planning to leave the profession in the next 4 years (White, 1998). These figures appear to reflect a growing disillusionment within the profession which stems from excessive workloads, high stress levels and recent controversial cuts in the service (Martell, 1998). Furthermore, over recent years, the health visiting service has been severely criticised for its universal approach and failure to target needs (Audit Commission, 1994; Roberts *et al.*, 1996). To counteract this, the use of clinical guidelines has been encouraged by a policy emphasis on specifying needs for which families are to be targeted (Audit Commission, 1994). A response to this has been the fact that many community Trusts now issue health visiting staff with practice guidelines to assist them in identifying vulnerable families, that is, those families who require greater input than that offered through the review process of the child health promotion programme (Hall, 1996). Furthermore, in an attempt to reduce home visiting time by health visitors, visiting protocols prescribing the numbers of home visits and/or client contacts that health visitors should be making with clients with children under school age are being widely introduced (Carney *et al.*, 1996).

In view of the difficulties facing health visiting, there is an urgent need to identify suitable criteria for use in service contracts with local commissioners. With the introduction of Primary Care Group commissioning, it is crucial that health visitors can articulate their practice and vindicate their role. As Rowe (1997: 288) has recently stated, 'the fact is there are lots of people... who don't know what health visitors and school nurses do'. Indeed, managers are continually faced with difficulties in making health visitor work practices explicit to purchasers; clinical guidelines are viewed by many as the way forward despite few efforts having been made to evaluate their effectiveness in practice. In view of the current interest in clinical practice guidelines, it seemed pertinent to undertake a study to assess the extent to which clinical guidelines are issued to health visitors working in England to assist them in identifying families requiring extra health visiting support and to examine their validity and reliability.

The study of practice guidelines

The study involved a national postal survey of the senior nurses of all 179 community Trusts in England employing health visiting staff. The survey had two purposes. The first was to gather information about the existence of clinical guidelines to assist health visitors in identifying and prioritising families needing extra health visiting support. Second, copies of local Trust guidelines were requested from each senior nurse, the intention being to examine the documents in order to evaluate their validity and reliability. The overall aim of the research was to build up a national picture of the existence of such guidelines in England for the identification of vulnerable children and families requiring increased health visitor intervention and support.

A postal questionnaire was developed and distributed to all community NHS Trust senior nurses employing health visitors. A complete list of senior nurses was obtained using an up-to-date NHS directory (*Binley's Directory of NHS Management*, 1994). This enabled the researcher to make direct contact with the sample population personally in writing. By targeting the total population of senior nurses, it was hoped to achieve a representative and unbiased sample. For this reason, a number of strategies were employed to try to enhance uptake as postal questionnaires can be problematic and are notorious for their low response rates (Scott, 1961; Moser and Kalton, 1971; Oppenheim, 1992; Polit and Hungler, 1994). The questionnaire was accompanied by a covering letter addressed to each senior nurse in person, detailing the nature of the research study, explaining the selection process and inviting participation in the project. Both Oppenheim (1992) and Newell (1993) have suggested that addressing envelopes and letters personally to the individual in question can help to increase response rates.

The questionnaire itself was a fairly short, two-sided document consisting of a combination of pre-coded closed questions and open-ended questions/statements. It was conservative in appearance, and a stamped addressed envelope was enclosed for ease of return. The main advantage of using a postal questionnaire in this study was that it is a fairly cheap method for gathering data and required a lot less time and energy to administer than interviews. These were important considerations for the researcher as the study formed the preliminary phase of a larger research project. It also enabled a large sample spread across the country to be targeted fairly easily. Other strategies, for example responding promptly to all telephone calls and requests for information or duplicate questionnaires, were also used to improve response rates. Each questionnaire was also office coded so that non-respondents could be followed up. Scott (1961: 164) argues that 'the use of follow-ups, or reminders, is certainly the most potent technique yet discovered for increasing the response rate'. The accompanying letter also encouraged the senior nurses to include copies of local clinical guidelines and policies when returning their questionnaire response.

A log of returned questionnaires was maintained throughout data collection. Three sets of data were generated:

1. The quantitative data generated through the closed questions/statements in the questionnaire were coded by hand and then entered onto the statistical package MINITAB (1991) and analysed descriptively.
2. The qualitative data from the two open-ended questions on the questionnaire were analysed using a simple process of qualitative content analysis.
3. The documents and guidelines for identifying and prioritising vulnerable families were critiqued as if they were research instruments in their own right. As no suitable tool was available to analyse the documents, a critique and analysis instrument was developed for use in the study.

Using documents in a research study

Researchers often overlook the potential wealth of information that can be gathered from existing records and documents, and many novice researchers fall into the trap of thinking that they must always set out to collect 'new'

data. Indeed, nursing records, protocols and clinical guidelines can provide community nurse researchers with easily
accessible and readily available research data. Using this
type of material in a research study means that the documents are recorded as secondary data sources because they
contain material 'not specifically gathered for the research
question at hand' (Stewart, 1984: 11). This differs from
the collection of primary research data, in which the
researcher is responsible for the entire research process
from the design of the project to collecting, analysing and
discussing the research data (Stewart, 1984).

The main advantages of using existing records/docu-
ments/clinical practice guidelines in a research study are that
the data are readily available, take little time to collect and
provide a relatively inexpensive form of information (Bailey,
1982; Treece and Treece, 1982; Webb *et al.*, 1984; Lincoln
and Guba, 1985; Polit and Hungler, 1994). This is often an
important consideration for community nurse researchers,
who may have little time allocated for research purposes. A
further strength of the use of documentary evidence is its
'non-reactivity' (Webb *et al.*, 1984: 114) – the fact that records
tend to be unbiased as the documents are usually collated
for other purposes. The researcher is not in a position to
bias subjects, and the authors of documents are unlikely to
assume their future use in research studies. Another advantage is the fact that the researcher can obtain data without
being 'present' in the field; this was demonstrated in the
present study, where documents were requested from Trust
senior nurses via the use of a questionnaire.

The disadvantages of documentary data also need highlighting (Bailey, 1982; Treece and Treece, 1982; Stewart,
1984; Webb *et al.*, 1984; While, 1987; Hakim, 1993; Appleton
and Cowley, 1997). Documentary analysis is limited by the
availability of material, missing or incomplete data, inac-
curacies in material and inherent biases. Webb *et al.* (1984:
114) identify the major sources of bias in documentary
evidence when they describe the two problems of 'selective survival' and 'selective deposit'. 'Selective survival'
(Webb *et al.*, 1984: 114) refers to missing or incomplete
data; 'relevant data may be censored for confidentiality

reasons' (Hakim, 1993: 136) or because their content may be perceived as reflecting badly on the institution/organisation (Webb *et al.*, 1984). Selective deposit refers to the representativeness of the sample.

Further difficulties can arise with the analysis of documentary research data. First are the difficulties inherent in being sure that the documents sent by organisations reflect the total document rather than just 'part' of an official document. Second, when analysing documents taken out of context, information contained within them may lack the clarification from associated training sessions. Third, documentary data, because they are presented in word form, usually demand much preparatory work before analysis can take place. This problem is magnified when documents lack a standard format. Finally, an obvious limitation of the study is the fact that documentary analysis can focus only on the existence and nature of guidelines as reported by senior nurses and cannot comment on health visitors' adherence to the guidelines in practice.

The critique and analysis tool

A number of researchers have highlighted the difficulties associated with the content analysis of documents, particularly the coding difficulties encountered when faced with a large number of documents that lack any standard format (Guba and Lincoln, 1981; Bailey, 1982; Treece and Treece, 1982; Hakim, 1993). As no suitable tool was available, a critique and analysis tool was developed to examine the 77 documents sent to the researcher. It is suggested that this instrument could be adapted for use in future research studies to evaluate the validity and reliability of clinical practice guidelines used in community nursing. For the purpose of the analysis, each document has been regarded as a 'research instrument'. The critique tool developed was informed by a number of texts but has been adapted primarily from the work of Guba and Lincoln (1981), Bailey (1982) and Treece and Treece (1982). The focus of the critique tool was to determine the nature of each document and to see whether the document could stand up to simple tests of reliability and validity, taking into consideration the reasons for the researcher undertaking this documentary analysis:

- to evaluate existing documents in order to describe their nature and content;
- to consider what underlying assumptions the documents made about the nature of 'vulnerability' and families requiring increased health visitor support;
- to analyse the indices/concepts/risk factors represented in the documents in order to examine how far they were supported by research evidence;
- to consider how well supported by research were the approaches that health visitors had taken to identify vulnerable families;
- to consider whether the clinical guidelines were intended as an aid to or a replacement for professional judgement.

The document analysis and critique tool (Figure 4.1) that was developed for use in this study was based on a 'checklist' of 38 questions/statements developed to be applied to each of the 77 documents. These questions were split into five separate sections within the critique tool. The purpose of the five parts of the critique and analysis tool will now be explored further.

Critique Questions	Comments
Part A – Authorship and body	
1. Questionnaire and document number	Office code for document
2. Authorship	
3. What is its origin? (For example, is there any evidence that indicates how the instrument was developed?	
4. What guidelines have been sent to the researcher?	
5. What focus do the vulnerability guidelines take?	
6. How are the guidelines formulated?	
7. Length of the document	
8. Do any instructions accompany the guidelines/checklist/document?	
9. Are the instructions clearly defined?	
10. How are assessment data recorded by the health visitors?	
Part B – Family vulnerability	
11. What is the stated function of the guidelines?	
12. What underlying assumptions are made about 'vulnerability' and families seen to be requiring increased health visitor support?	
13. Is family vulnerability linked with child protection?	
14. Do the guidelines recognise that vulnerability is a complex, ambiguous and transient concept?	
15. Do the assumptions upon which the guidelines are based serve to clarify and/or help to stabilise the nature of vulnerability, or negate it by failing to recognise the embedded complexities?	
Part C – Professional judgement	
16. Is professional judgement valued?	
17. If it is valued, at what level is it valued?	
18. Does professional judgement stand alone?	

19. Do the guidelines aid professional judgement?		
20. Is professional judgement tagged on as an afterthought? (For example, a sort of let-out clause?)		
21. What appears to be the relative importance of 'professional judgements' to the guidelines?		
Part D – Reliability and validity		
22. Do the documents/guidelines provide any evidence of reliability?		
23. Are there any errors in the instruments? If yes, what?		
24. Internal consistency: how clearly detailed and defined are the indices?		
25. Are all the indices on the instrument measuring the same thing?		
26. How have they been sampled?		
27. Equivalence: Have any of the following issues been considered? (For example, training for health visitor users of the instrument, inconsistencies between health visitors using the instrument, health visitor bias, standardised measurement schedule and so on)		
28. Do the documents/guidelines provide any evidence of validity?		
29. Do all the indices deal with vulnerability?		
30. Has the content of the instrument been judged to be appropriate?		
31. Are the indices robust? (For example, can they stand alone? Are they independent? Are they valid concepts?)		
32. What research evidence supports the validity of the indices?		
33. How successfully have the concepts been operationalised? (For example, are each of the indices/concepts identified measuring the concept they were designed to measure?)		
34. Are the indices accepted measures? If so, why?		
35. How clearly detailed and defined are the indices?		
36. Is the 'halo effect' in operation?		
37. Is the health visitor required to make a forced choice?		
Part E – Risk factors /risk indices		
38. List of risk factors/risk indices		

Figure 4.1 Critique and analysis tool for documents

Part A – Authorship and body

The aim of part A was to obtain a broad overview of the nature of each document/research instrument. Each document was logged according to its office code number (statement 1). This section of the critique tool focuses mainly on 'Authorship – who conceived the material?' and 'Body – the form on which the data are found' (Treece and Treece, 1982: 268). Questions were raised about whether any instructions accompanied the guidelines/document as this could influence reliability. One question focused on how and where assessment data were recorded by health visitors using the research instrument.

Part B – Family vulnerability

The second section of the critique and analysis tool centred on the concept of 'vulnerability' and increased support offered to vulnerable families by health visitors. The five questions in this section concentrated on the stated 'Function – the purpose or reason' (Treece and Treece, 1982: 268) for the guidelines. Question 12 explored what underlying assumptions are made about 'vulnerability' and families seen to be requiring increased health visitor support. In view of previous research findings (Appleton, 1994), it appeared to be important to determine whether or not the guidelines recognised vulnerability as a complex, ambiguous and transient concept. Exploring whether family vulnerability and hence increased health visitor support were linked with child protection was also addressed. This was because an earlier review of the literature (Appleton, 1994) indicated that the majority of studies in which health visitors have been involved in making assessments of vulnerable families have tended to focus on the use of screening procedures for families 'at risk' of child abuse.

Part C – Professional judgement

This section considered professional judgement and decision-making skills. Questions in this section were planned to elicit detail about professional decisions and the relationship between official guidelines and professional judgements. This appeared highly pertinent in view of the fact that a recent review of the literature had revealed that the majority of research studies in which health visitors had been involved in making assessments of vulnerable families included the use of checklists or screening tools rather than an evaluation of the health visitors' own assessment processes. Research evidence also seems to suggest that health visitors rely on their own professional judgements rather than on guidance from official guidelines in the assessment of vulnerable families (Appleton, 1993; Williams, 1997).

Part D – Reliability and validity

This section of the critique and analysis tool concentrated on the research basis of the guidelines. Initial questions focused on the reliability of the documents and 'the extent to which a measure gives consistent results' (Nolan and Behi, 1995a: 472). Three aspects of reliability are usually explored when studying the reliability of a measuring instrument:

- internal consistency
- stability
- equivalence.

Internal consistency, 'the extent to which all the instrument's subparts or items are measuring the same attribute' (Polit and Hungler, 1994: 386) was considered first in the critique tool. To estimate internal consistency, the researcher had to consider whether all the indices on the instrument were in fact measuring the same concept. It was therefore important to consider how clearly detailed and defined were the indices within the documents and to consider how they had been sampled.

The stability of a measure 'refers to the extent to which the same results are obtained on repeated administrations of the instrument. Estimation of reliability here focuses on the instrument's susceptibility to extraneous factors from one administration to the next' (Polit and Hungler, 1994: 368). The researcher felt that it was inappropriate to consider the 'stability' of the documents sent as no test/retest measurement facility existed. However, it is probable that fluctuations in measurement will occur over a period of time because of the nature of what is being measured, that is, the need for families to receive increased health visitor support. For this reason alone, instruments are likely to show low reliability.

The third aspect of reliability that was considered in relation to the documents was 'equivalence'. 'Equivalence' is the extent to which different health visitors using the same instrument applied to the same individual or family at the same time, or when two parallel instruments are applied to the same individual or family at the same time, obtain consistent results (Reardon-Castles, 1987; Polit and Hungler, 1994). This is commonly known as interrater reliability. In terms of the equivalence of the health visitor documents, the researcher considered whether the following issues had been addressed:

- training for users of the instrument;
- the competency and ability of the health visitors;
- inconsistencies between health visitors using the instrument;
- health visitor bias;
- a standardised measurement scale to reduce the risk of bias.

It is, however, important to recognise that just because a document did not actually mention training for users of the instrument, this does not mean that training did not occur in practice in the Trusts. This illustrates one of the disadvantages highlighted earlier of 'incomplete data', which can be problematic when analysing documents.

Evidence of validity was also considered in this section of the critique tool. Validity is 'the degree to which an instrument measures what it is intended to measure' (Polit and Hungler, 1994: 657). The validity of a measure (Bowling, 1991; LoBiondo-Wood and Haber, 1994; Polit and Hungler, 1994; Nolan and Behi, 1995b) is usually considered in terms of:

1. face validity;
2. content validity;
3. criterion-related validity, which is differentiated as:
   • concurrent validity
   • predictive validity
   • construct validity.

Face validity is the weakest form of validity and is usually regarded as a highly subjective measure (Treece and Treece, 1982; Reardon-Castles, 1987). Within the critique tool, face validity was addressed by critically examining each document and considering whether all the items included dealt with vulnerability and appeared to measure families requiring increased support from health visitors. To estimate content validity, the researcher considered whether the content of the documents had been judged to be appropriate for the purposes of the document (Treece and Treece, 1982; Gibbon, 1995). The content of a document may be judged to be appropriate if a literature review has been undertaken that informs and supports its content. Pilot work may have been completed to assess the representativeness of the document's content, or a group of experts may have been consulted about the items included within a document, particularly the risk indices incorporated in an official guideline (Treece and Treece, 1982; Burns and Grove, 1997).

It was not feasible to address criterion-related validity when analysing the documents. This is because both concurrent and predictive validity involve the measure being correlated with some external criterion (standard/instrument), which has already been judged to be valid (Powers and Knapp, 1990). The author is not aware of any clinical guideline issued to health visitors to assist them in the identification of families requiring increased support that has been proved to be truly valid and reliable.

Construct validity refers 'to the validity of the theory behind the [measure]' (Herbert, 1990: 3) and is considered to be the most important aspect of validity. Construct validity in relation to the documents is concerned with the extent to which the results of applying the documents reflect the underlying theoretical concepts, the vulnerability indices. This would be 'the extent to which the theoretical concepts have been successfully operationalised' (Herbert, 1990: 17). In terms of the vulnerability indices, the researcher considered whether they were accepted measures, whether or not the indices were robust and valid concepts, and what research evidence supported this. Questions were also raised regarding how the concepts were detailed and defined; this is important to ensure that the same meaning is shared by health visitors in order to reduce the risk of bias.

Part E – Risk factors/risk indices

The final section of the critique tool listed and coded all the risk factors/indices mentioned in each document.

Analysing the documentary data

Having developed the critique and analysis tool for the documents, a computer database was established using Microsoft Excel. Reviewing each document and registering information on the database was a time-consuming and laborious process. However, consolidating the documentary data on Microsoft Excel enabled pertinent issues to be explored more easily, which is particularly important when dealing with documents of different formats and lengths.

The qualitative documentary data (questions 2–37) were analysed question by question separately for words, descriptions and recurrent categories. Diagrams were then constructed to illustrate in visual form how the categories linked together. The data were continually compared with the associated questionnaire data. The listed risk factors/indices (question 38 onwards) were analysed using a simple quantitative enumeration approach, which was helpful in illustrating the range of risk factors contained in the documents, exploring the frequency with which they were cited and examining the research evidence supporting their use in the guidelines.

Findings

Following a 3-month period of data collection, the exploratory questionnaire resulted in a response rate of 87 per cent (156 senior nurses). There was clearly much interest in the topic, and this was further supported by the fact that nearly 60 per cent of areas were willing to allow health visitors in their Trust to participate further in the study. Of the 98 (63.2 per cent) senior nurses stating that their Trusts had official guidelines to assist health visitors in identifying and prioritising vulnerable families, 67 (68.37 per cent) areas enclosed a copy of the guidelines. Indeed, eight Trusts sent copies of two different types of guideline that they distributed to staff, and one area sent three, so altogether a total of 77 separate guidelines was received.

Nature of existing guidelines

Many of the guidelines sent were presented as formal protocols and, quite significantly, there was a lack of uniformity between them. The majority of documents – 35 (45.45 per cent) – were classified as checklists, scoring systems and screening tools that appeared to be heavily influenced by the scoring approaches of non-health visitors used in screening for risk assessment in child abuse (Appleton, 1997).

Reliability of guidelines

Each guideline was critically examined to determine evidence of validity and reliability. Overall, the guidelines provided little evidence of reliability. There was a lack of structured assessment format that could reduce the risk of user bias, and many of the risk indices identified in the guidelines were fairly subjective in nature and not well defined. The reliance on professional opinion of concerns undoubtedly allows a different emphasis to be placed on each specific aspect of the assessment, and this level of subjectivity was highlighted by a number of respondents.

The maze of risk indices

Many of the guidelines included risk factors/risk indices in some form. When all the various indices/risk factors were collated, there were 133 different types mentioned in the documents, many of which were not supported by sound research evidence. The 11 most frequently cited risk indices are highlighted in Table 4.1 below.

Table 4.1   The most frequently cited risk indices

Risk factors/indices	Frequency
Mental health problems	60
Chronic illness, birth defect or development lag	56
Unrealistic expectations of child and generally negative attitude to child	49
Abuse of alcohol and/or drugs	49
Chronic illness/health problems	48
Social/economic problems	48
Substandard living conditions	45
Poor extended family relationships/isolation	44
Poor parenting affecting the child's health	44
Known to be violent and/or suicidal	41
Below 20 (or other specified age) at birth of first child	41

The documents provided little evidence of internal consistency as in 55 (80.88 per cent) of the 68 guidelines that included risk factors or listed indices in some form, indices were included that were not defined in detail. For example, most indices are only one or a few words long: Q.457 refers to 'single parents' and 'poverty', Q.917 'birth trauma' and 'poor housing', and Q.764 'parenting skills', 'medical' and 'social'. These terms are all open to varied interpretations by different health visitors; their vagueness and lack of specificity reduce the reliability of the measuring instruments. The majority of community Trusts – 62 (80.52 per cent) – gave no indication of how the content of the guidelines had been sampled. Over two-thirds of the guidelines – 55 (71.43 per cent) – provided no evidence of equivalence, giving no information about training for users of the instrument, the competency and ability of the health visitors, inconsistencies between health visitors using the instrument and health visitor bias.

Reliability was addressed in a small number of guidelines in which the health visitors were encouraged to discuss a family that was causing them concern with a nurse advisor/manager and in which staff using the guideline undertook an associated training session.

Validity of guidelines

Within the critique tool, face validity was addressed by critically reviewing each document and considering whether all the items included dealt with vulnerability and appeared to measure families requiring increased support from health visitors. Most of the guidelines – 54 out of 68 (79.41 per cent) – that included risk indices in some form gave equal weighting to all risk indices. Thus, in guideline 317, 'unusual forename' was given an equal weighting to 'previous history of family violence or child abuse'. A number of guidelines clearly did not recognise that family vulnerability could be the result of multiple interacting factors, some guidelines focusing solely on certain aspects, such as the child or parent/carer, with none of the suggested indices focusing on wider social, cultural, environmental or emotional issues.

Content validity was assessed by determining whether the content of the documents had been judged to be appropriate for the purposes of the guideline (Treece and Treece, 1982; Gibbon, 1995). Grimshaw and Russell (1993) have stressed the importance of assessing the validity of a clinical guideline by determining whether there is evidence of a formal systematic literature review having been completed. However, only 8 (8.16 per cent) of the 98 respondents who stated that guidelines were available in their Trust commented on having undertaken a literature review, and questions can be raised about the effectiveness of the reviews completed. Indeed, an in-depth review would have determined that although a number of research studies have focused on risk assessment in terms of child protection, many of the tools/guidelines used in previous health visiting studies lack validity and/or have not been evaluated properly (Hills *et al.*, 1980; Woods, 1981; Fort, 1986; Browne, 1995; Walker and Crapper, 1995).

Guidelines and service contracts

In view of the ongoing government emphasis on a more effective and efficient use of existing NHS resources, it appeared important to consider whether and how managers were marketing health visiting services with vulnerable families. Two recent NHS Executive documents have also recommended that guidelines should be used to 'inform contracts' (NHSME, 1993; NHSE, 1994). Thus, respondents were asked about whether or not 'vulnerability' guidelines entered into contracting arrangements between purchasers and providers. Currently, only a small number of community Trusts 35 (35.71 per cent) include the clinical practice guidelines to assist health visitors in identifying vulnerable families in service contracts. However, many areas were addressing the issue and considering the need to include the guidelines in contracts in the future. It is worrying that many Trusts are considering the inclusion of clinical guidelines to assist health visitors in identifying vulnerable families in service contracts when the majority appear to lack validity and reliability. A problem with rigid adherence to clinical practice guidelines is that vulnerable families could be missed and important preventive work not be undertaken.

The research basis of guidelines

Of the 98 community Trusts issuing guidelines to assist health visitors in identifying and prioritising vulnerable families, only 19 (19.39 per cent) respondents who stated that the guidelines were based on published research were able to refer to a published study. The majority of research studies – 17 (89.47 per cent) – to which respondents referred are studies related to screening for potential child abuse. This indicates that there appears to be a strong link between child protection and the respondents' perceptions of guidelines to assist health visitors in making assessments of families needing extra intervention. This is further supported by the fact that the documentary analysis also revealed that in 33 (42.86 per cent) cases, the documents issued to health visitors to assist them in identifying vulnerable families were closely linked to child protection.

Eleven comments were made about studies not directly relevant to child protection; this could indicate a recognition by some community NHS Trusts that families may be 'vulnerable' and in need of increased health visitor support for reasons other than child protection concerns. Of the 11, 4 (36.36 per cent) referred to sudden infant death syndrome/Care Of Next Infant (CONI) research and 3 (27.27 per cent) to the Edinburgh Postnatal Depression research. Both schemes are closely linked with increased support from the health visiting service.

Interestingly, the majority of questionnaire respondents attempted to discuss research in a non-specific and rather vague manner. Being optimistic, this could mean that there is a research basis to the guidelines but that the respondents are not able to articulate it. However, the present situation appeared to be summed up by one respondent who stated:

The vulnerability indices... enclosed have been gobbled (sic) together to at least give health visitors a means of making some decisions. They are warned that they are indices only and not entirely infallible. (Q.734.)

Overall, the research-based evidence supporting the use of guidelines to assist health visitors in identifying and prioritising families is minimal. Furthermore, the fact that many of the documents sent to the researcher are not based on systematic research reviews raises the question of whether they should really be regarded as 'clinical practice guidelines' at all (Grimshaw and Russell, 1993; Nuffield Institute for Health, 1994). Perhaps 'local guideline' is a more accurate description for these types of documents.

Professional judgement and practice implications

Despite the wide variation in clinical guidelines in existence or sent to the researcher, it was interesting to find that professional judgement was recognised in 33 (42.86 per cent) of the guidelines to some extent and appeared to be implicit in another 20 (25.97 per cent). Thus, a total of 53 (68.83 per cent) guidelines to some extent recognised the importance of professional judgement . Evidently, further research is needed to explore clinical decision-making in health visiting, particularly in terms of identifying families needing increased interventions. There are clearly a number of pertinent issues here:

- Does the use of checklists and guidelines constrain professional judgement?
- To what extent do assessment guidelines and visiting protocols direct health visitors in making assessments of family health needs?
- Do health visitors make their own clinical assessments of families needing extra support or do they have a checklist at the back of their mind or a guideline to refer to?
- Are newly qualified staff more likely to make use of official guidelines than more experienced staff?

If health visitors are using their professional judgements to make family assessments (and within many guidelines, professional judgement can stand alone), this raises the important issue of whether health visitors should be exerting influence on managers not to rely on dubious checklists or guidelines. Furthermore, senior nurses in 57 (36.8 per cent) community Trusts stated that no clinical guidelines were issued to health visitors, and one would assume that health visitors in these areas are relying on their own professional judgements to make family assessments. There is clearly an urgent need for professional judgement in health visiting practice to be explored further and the processes involved in clinical decision-making to be detailed and examined.

Conclusion

Documentary evidence can provide the researcher with a wealth of rich and detailed data that is unbiased by the data collection process. This chapter has described the processes undertaken when developing a method for the data analysis of clinical guidelines used in health visiting practice to identify families needing increased support. In view of the recent concerns raised by the Royal College of Nursing (RCN) (1995) and Hutchinson *et al.* (1995) about clinical guidelines, it is essential that community nurses start to consider the validity and relevance of clinical practice guidelines used in health visiting practice. Practitioners need to consider whether the use of clinical guidelines could constrain professional practice and examine the legal and ethical implications surrounding their use. It is also important to question whether it is ever appropriate to attempt to replace professional judgement, as suggested by the shift towards the greater use of clinical guidelines in contract specifications.

The documentary analysis method described in this chapter has revealed evidence that formal, but generally subjective and invalid, guidelines are widely in existence throughout the country for identifying families with increased health/

social needs. Maybe it is time for health visitors and community nurse managers to heed the warning of Grimshaw and Russell (1993: 245), who state that 'if those developing guidelines fail to overcome the many potential biases inherent in that development, the resulting guidelines may recommend ineffective or even dangerous clinical practice'.

KEY POINTS

■ Existing records, documents and clinical guidelines offer a wealth of rich data for community nurse researchers.

■ Where clinical guidelines are currently in existence in community nursing to search for health needs, practitioners need to evaluate the guidelines' validity and reliability, and establish whether they are based on sound research evidence.

■ Many of the guidelines in existence to assist health visitors in the identification of families requiring extra health visiting support lack validity and reliability, and provide very limited supporting research evidence.

■ A worrying feature is the increasing use of clinical guidelines in contract specifications when they may not reflect actual practice.

■ The nature and value of health visitors' professional judgements in identifying health needs should be examined in more detail and the factors that influence those judgements explicated.

Acknowledgement

Many thanks to all the senior nurses who participated in this phase of the study.

References

Antrobus S. and Brown S. (1996) Guidelines and protocols: a chance to take the lead. *Nursing Times* **92**(23): 38–9.

Appleton J.V. (1993) An Exploratory Study of the Health Visitor's Role in Identifying and Working with Vulnerable Families in Relation to Child Protection. Unpublished MSc thesis, King's College London, University of London.

Appleton J.V. (1994) The concept of vulnerability in relation to child protection; health visitors' perceptions. *Journal of Advanced Nursing* **20**: 1132–40.

Appleton J.V. (1997) Establishing the validity and reliability of clinical practice guidelines used to identify families requiring increased health visitor support. *Public Health* **111**: 107–13.

Appleton J.V. and Cowley S. (1997) Analysing clinical practice guidelines. A method of documentary analysis. *Journal of Advanced Nursing* **25**: 1008–17.

Audit Commission (1994) *Seen but not Heard.* London: HMSO.

Bailey K.D. (1982) *Methods of Social Research*, (2nd edn). New York: Free Press.

Binley's Directory of NHS Management (1994) Essex: Beechwood House.

Bowling A. (1991) *Measuring Health: A Review of Quality of Life Measures.* Buckingham: Open University Press.

Browne K. (1995) Preventing child maltreatment through community nursing. *Journal of Advanced Nursing* **21**: 57–63.

Burns N. and Grove S.K. (1997) *The Practice of Nursing Research. Conduct, Critique and Utilization*, (3rd edn). Philadelphia: W.B. Saunders.

Carney O., McIntosh J., Worth A. and Lugton J. (1996) Assessment of need for health visiting. Research Monograph No.2. Glasgow: Department of Nursing and Community Health, Glasgow Caledonian University.

Carruthers I. (1995) Clinical guidelines: a health commission perspective. In Deighan M. and Hitch S. (eds) *Clinical Effectiveness from Guidelines to Cost-effective Practice.* Brentwood: Earlybrave Publications/Health Services Management Unit.

Deighan M. and Hitch S. (eds) (1995) *Clinical Effectiveness from Guidelines to Cost-effective Practice.* Brentwood: Earlybrave Publications/Health Services Management Unit.

Duff L.A., Kitson A.L., Seers K. and Humphris D. (1996) Clinical guidelines: an introduction to their development and implementation. *Journal of Advanced Nursing* **23**: 887–95.

Eddy D.M. (1990) Practice policies – what are they? *Journal of the American Medical Association* **263**: 877–80.

Field M.J. and Lohr K.N. (1992) *Guidelines for Clinical Practice. From Development to Use.* Washington, DC: National Academy Press.

Fort A. (1986) The spider's web. *Health Service Journal* **96**: 558–9.

Gibbon B. (1995) Validity and reliability of assessment tools. *Nurse Researcher* **2**(2): 48–55.

Grimshaw J. and Russell I. (1993) Achieving health gain through clinical guidelines. I: Developing scientifically valid guidelines. *Quality in Health Care* **2**: 243–8.

Guba E.G. and Lincoln Y.S. (1981) *Effective Evaluation.* San Francisco, CA: Jossey-Bass.

Hakim C. (1993) Research analysis of administrative records. In Hammersley M. (ed.) *Social Research, Philosophy, Politics and Practice.* London: Sage.

Hall D.M.B. (1996) *Health for all Children* (3rd edn). Oxford: Oxford University Press.

Health Visitors' Association (HVA) (1994) *A Cause for Concern: An Analysis of Staffing Levels and Training Plans in Health Visiting and School Nursing.* London: HVA.

Herbert M. (1990) *Planning a Research Project. A Guide for Practitioners and Trainees in the Helping Professions.* London: Cassell.

Hills A., Parson S.A. and Turner B. (1980) Health visiting priorities. *Nursing Times (Community Outlook)* **10**: 295–9.

Hutchinson A., McIntosh A., Roberts A. and Sutton P. (1995) Evidence based health care: the challenge for general practice. In Deighan M. and Hitch S. (eds) *Clinical Effectiveness from Guidelines to Cost-effective Practice.* Brentwood: Earlybrave Publications/ Health Services Management Unit.

Klazinga N. (1995) Clinical guidelines bridging evidence based medicine and health services reform: a European perspective. In Deighan M. and Hitch S. (eds) *Clinical Effectiveness from Guidelines to Cost-effective Practice.* Brentwood: Earlybrave Publications/Health Services Management Unit.

Lincoln Y.S. and Guba E.G. (1985) *Naturalistic Inquiry.* California: Sage.

Lobiondo-Wood G. and Haber J. (1994) *Nursing Research: Methods, Critical Appraisal and Utilisation.* St Louis: C.V. Mosby.

Martell R. (1998) Community cuts have 'devastated' basic services. *Nursing Times* **94**(39): 7.

MINITAB (1991) Minitab Statistical Software. Cle.com, Birmingham: Minitab Inc.

Moser C.A. and Kalton G. (1971) *Survey Methods in Social Investigation.* Aldershot: Gower.

Newell R. (1993) Sampling and distribution issues. *Nurse Researcher* **1**(2): 33–43.

NHS Management Executive (NHSME) (1993) *Improving Clinical Effectiveness.* EL 115. Leeds: DoH.

NHS Executive (NHSE) (1994) *Improving the Effectiveness of the NHS.* EL 74. Leeds: DoH.

Nolan M. and Behi R. (1995a) Reliability: consistency and accuracy in measurement. *British Journal of Nursing* **4**(5): 472–5.

Nolan M. and Behi R. (1995b) Validity: a concept at the heart of research. *British Journal of Nursing* **4**(9): 530–3.

Nuffield Institute for Health (1994) *Effective Health Care: Implementing Clinical Practice Guidelines: Can Guidelines be Used to Improve Clinical Practice?* Bulletin No. 8. Leeds: University of Leeds.

Oppenheim A.N. (1992) *Questionnaire Design, Interviewing and Attitude Measurement.* London: Pinter Publishers.

Polit D.F. and Hungler B.P. (1994) *Nursing Research. Principles and Methods* (5th edn). Philadelphia: J.B. Lippincott.

Powers B.A. and Knapp T.R. (1990) *A Dictionary of Nursing Theory and Research.* California: Sage.

Reardon-Castles M. (1987) *Primer of Nursing Research.* Philadelphia: W.B. Saunders.

Roberts C. *et al.* (1996) The proof of the pudding. *Health Service Journal* **106**(5494): 27.

Rowe J. (1997) Cited in Cole A., Buying time. *Health Visitor* **70**(8): 287–8.

Royal College of Nursing (RCN) (1995) *Research Society Newsletter. Clinical Guidelines.* (Sept): 16–18.

Russell I. and Grimshaw J. (1995) Health technology assessment: basis of valid guidelines *and* test of effective implementation? In Deighan M. and Hitch S. (eds) *Clinical Effectiveness from Guidelines to Cost-effective Practice.* Brentwood: Earlybrave Publications/Health Services Management Unit.

Sackett D. and Rosenberg W. (1995) Evidence-based medicine & guidelines. In Deighan M. and Hitch S. (eds) *Clinical Effectiveness from Guidelines to Cost-effective Practice.* Brentwood: Earlybrave Publications/Health Services Management Unit.

Sackett D.L., Rosenberg W.M., Gray J.A., Haynes R.B. and Richardson W.S. (1996) Evidence based medicine: what it is and what it isn't. *British Medical Journal* **312**(7023): 71–2 (editorial).

Scott C. (1961) Research on mail surveys. *Journal of the Royal Statistical Society Series (A)* **124**(2): 143–205.

Stewart D.W. (1984) *Secondary Research. Information Sources and Methods.* Newbury Park, CA: Sage.

Sullivan J.M. and Mann R.J. (1994) Clinical practice guidelines: implications for use. *Dermatology Nursing* **6**(6): 413–18.

Treece E.W. and Treece J.W. (1982) *Elements of Research in Nursing* (3rd edn). St Louis: C.V. Mosby.

Von Degenberg K. (1996) An effective health service: can it be achieved? *Nursing Times Research* **1**(5): 340–6.

Walker M. and Crapper E. (1995) Identifying families of concern. *Primary Health Care* **5**(2): 12–14.

Webb E.J., Campbell D.T., Schwarz R.D. and Sechrest L. (1984) The use of archival sources in social research. In Bulmer M. (ed.) *Sociological Research Methods – an Introduction.* London: Macmillan.

While A.E. (1987) Records as a data source: the case for health visitor records. *Journal of Advanced Nursing* **12**: 757–63.

White C. (1998) Crisis in health visiting as staff disillusionment grows. *Nursing Times* **94**(42): 6.
Williams D.M. (1977) Vulnerable families: a study of health visitors' prioritization of their work. *Journal of Nursing Management* **5**: 19–24.
Woods J. (1981) A practical approach to preventing child abuse. *Health Visitor* **54**: 281–3.

5

Lay Perspectives on Health Needs

Jenny Billings

The importance of including the perceived health needs and views of users of the health services has been well articulated within previous government policy (DoH, 1989, 1993; NHSME, 1991; NHSE, 1995) and among those concerned with obtaining client perceptions of health need, such as Bowling (1992) and Goodwin (1994). This opinion continues to be supported in the White Paper, *The New NHS* (DoH, 1997), which specifies that decisions about health care will be taken by newly formed Primary Health Care Groups close to the client so that health care provision can be purchased according to local needs. Lay representation on the boards of Primary Care Groups may also act as an important lever to enacting these policy requirements.

Despite the political emphasis, the issue of public participation in health care planning is not new. In a review by Cooper *et al.* (1995), there is evidence to suggest an extensive body of international literature on the subject dating back to the 1960s. The more recent 'Local Voices' initiative (NHSME, 1992) was instrumental in relaunching the movement in this country, containing as it did a powerful injunction to health authorities to engage seriously in public consultation. This exercise was seen as being vital to ensure that services were better suited to meeting the health needs of the local population and to encourage public support for any health care decisions made. Cooper *et al.* (1995) noted that the initiative resulted in a 'flurry' of published examples of projects, demonstrating that obtaining the consumer view was being addressed in one way or another by health authorities. Common methods included public meetings, focus groups, health forums, rapid appraisal, telephone hotlines, consumer satisfaction surveys, interviews and complaints procedures.

This desire to obtain the consumer view has been further fuelled by a growing criticism of the more traditional methods of assessing health needs within a population. The main arguments centre around a critique of the normative and professionally defined nature of epidemiological information, the measurement of pathology being central to the prioritisation of health services to the neglect of the lived experiences and perceived needs of the lay population (Peckham and Spanton, 1994; Billings, 1995). The increasing use of community health profiles, which are compiled using a more diverse range of health-related information, still tends to omit the consumer perceptions of need and focuses upon the more accessible epidemiology (Billings and Cowley, 1995; Billings, 1996). The resulting picture of health needs obtained using these methods will always be one of negative health states, failing perhaps to capture alternative health experiences.

Those who have embarked upon consumer perspective research have, however, encountered considerable difficulties in ensuring that health needs are represented. Richards (1991), for example, raises the question of how needs can be aggregated and synthesised into actual service provision. Bias may be an inevitable consequence as, despite the method used, it is often the middle classes whose needs are heard the most clearly during public consultation exercises unless care is taken to ensure appropriate representation from less advantaged groups (Rodgers, 1994). As a result, Stalker (1993) believes that there is the danger that 'felt' need can never be fully identified. Cooper *et al.* (1995) infer that the 'Local Voices' initiatives may be nothing more than tokenism, as health authorities have struggled with a singular lack of guidance to resolve the inevitable conflict between different health care provision viewpoints and available resources.

In a recent family health needs study conducted by Cowley and Billings (1997), the authors addressed these issues of data aggregation and the representation of consumer perceptions of health need in the first two phases of their study. These phases comprised a community profile and in-depth interviews with randomly selected clients from one GP practice. The authors developed a method of data analysis adapted from Yin's (1994) case study design, using a pattern-matching approach that allowed for a case description to emerge. The wider study was concerned with developing and purchasing services to meet the needs of families from a GP perspective and is documented elsewhere (Cowley and Billings, 1997). An overview of the method and first phase will be given, followed by a fuller account of the second phase.

Background: profiling

In the first phase of the study, a community profile was compiled consisting of data drawn from sources such as public health, housing, child health, child and family psychiatric services, local acute and community Trusts and the health authority. Local research studies and audits were also included. The following strategy was used to screen and aggregate the data:

1. Data sources were analysed according to their methodological requirements, and statistically available data were critically reviewed.
2. Themes relating to the identification of need were tabulated, enabling the emergence of patterns of need and links across data.
3. Data were organised on maps for further pattern-matching and 'goodness of fit'.
4. Emergent themes were matched with health theories and research to strengthen their position as indicators of need. (Yin, 1994)

In keeping with the use of largely normative data, the results provided a comparative picture of predominantly negative health in the population. A previous study in the area had highlighted high levels of deprivation and need within the local population (Cowley, 1991), and the pattern-matching allowed the extent of this deprivation to become explicit. Five major themes were identified, relating to mortality and morbidity, mental health, socioeconomic status, social housing and the health of children and young people. Within these categories, an incidence higher than the local or national average was identified for various health-related criteria. For example:

- The rate of heart disease, cancer and suicide was higher than local and national averages despite having a relatively younger population than neighbouring areas.
- At the time of the study, the rate of child abuse was much higher than the national average, and there was an 18-month waiting list for child and family psychiatric services.
- The town had some of the highest Jarman scores in the country (Jarman, 1984), a measure of the extent of deprivation and a trend of high long-term unemployment.

The second 'interview' phase of the project offered the opportunity to develop and test methods of fully blending client perceptions of need into the profile findings. Furthermore, one of the aims was to explore the extent to which the views of service users could influence local purchasing decisions. It was intended that interviews would potentially yield data that would be equally amenable to the pattern-matching approach in order to provide illustrations and perhaps tentative explanations of the patterns of ill health in the town developed from the profile information. This would in turn guide the development of new services. It was thus felt to be important to supplement the largely professionally defined information that was gathered from the community profile phase to this end, with a 'back to basics' look at the local perception of health need.

The interview schedule

An interview schedule was devised that would allow for the collection of quantitative and qualitative data in order to provide a picture of health need that was statistically comparable, as well as getting personal accounts of health. It was important to include some demographic details such as age, marital status, occupational class and housing so that the results could be compared with other health and social research such as that conducted by Graham (1984).

Previous analysis of the profile data in phase one of the project was valuable in highlighting key areas that influenced health both in the long and the short term. These areas were used as a basis for the content of the schedule and were formulated into questions about employment, housing, social support, childcare, physical and mental health, relationships, income and service provision. The schedule also contained the Edinburgh Postnatal Depression Scale (Cox *et al.*, 1987) and a self-esteem inventory (Rosenberg, 1965) to obtain a 'snapshot' view of the mental health status of respondents. It was considered appropriate to administer the Postnatal Depression Scale to mothers with children under one and the self-esteem inventory to those with older children. This is rationalised elsewhere (see Cowley and Billings, 1997).

It was appreciated that the use of themes predetermined by the profile data had the potential to perpetuate a negative orientation to health, so it was intended that the interview schedule would focus primarily on obtaining a health and well-being perspective rather than one focused on illness and morbidity. This approach centres on the salutogenic idea developed by Antonovsky (1987) and Cowley (1995) that health states are influenced by the availability of 'resources for health' and that these factors can optimise well-being. It was hoped that the respondents would reveal collectively tried and tested lay health strategies for coping. The eventual interview schedule was divided into two parts: a self-administered questionnaire for the collection of quantitative data comprised part 1, and part 2 consisted of prompts on a sheet of paper to guide a tape-recorded semi-structured interview.

Piloting

Piloting offered the opportunity for content, administrative and organisational issues to be assessed. The letter to be sent to respondents urging them to take part was given particular attention and was submitted to a range of mothers in a different area for their opinions on its readibility, comprehension and general layout.

Piloting is an often-neglected area of research but one vital for optimising recruitment; it also proved to be helpful with respect to deleting academic jargon. Pilot interviews with four families provided the opportunity to sharpen interview techniques in relation to monitoring the skills of reflection, summarising and clarification, as well as keeping some focus on such a broad topic area (Fontana and Frey, 1994). The pilot established that interviews could take any length of time, from 20 minutes to 2 hours, because of the diverse nature of people's experiences and their desire to relate them. Transcription was undertaken by a secretary.

Obtaining the sample

The initial plan was to select 100 families with children under 18 still in residence, using the statistical software package MINITAB to acquire a stratified random sample from the GP case list. A slight bias towards families with preschool children was allowed, reflecting research indicating their greater use of health services (Graham, 1994), 60 families with preschool children and 40 families with children aged 6–18 being selected.

Data collection started in November 1994. Respondents were contacted using the piloted letter with a choice of where the interview could take place (in their home or at the surgery). Included in the information was a stamped addressed envelope and a contact telephone number, allowing respondents the opportunity to confirm interviews by telephone or to change appointment times. If there was no reply after 2 weeks, a follow-up letter was sent out. It was intended that the main carer in each family would be the focus of the interview, in recognition of their central role in the family, as argued by Doyal (1983) and Graham (1987). The likelihood of the sample being largely composed of women was high, as authors such as Foster and Mayall (1990) state that women are still seen as the primary care-givers. In households where the care was said to be shared, or where the male partner was unemployed, the woman was still targeted. This is based on the rationale provided by Demi and Warren (1995), who have indicated that, in these situations, mothers are still largely responsible for family care and the management of the household, partners tending to assist.

Despite careful planning, it is often difficult to envisage the scale of the problems that may be encountered, particularly in relation to recruitment. It quickly became clear that the target of 100 interviews was overambitious as response rates were poor despite follow-up letters for those who had not replied. By the end of December, the response rate was 38.7 per cent, only 12 interviews having taken place. Table 5.1 summarises the recruitment after 2 months.

Table 5.1   Recruitment summary 2 months after commencement

Total sent out	Replies	Refusals	Interviews	Response rate (%)
31	12	6	13	38.7

Following a steering group meeting in January 1995, the following changes to the recruitment strategy were made:

- The original letter was altered, rendering it more informal. It was decided that postal recruitment would continue.
- A letter of endorsement from one of the GPs was drafted, encouraging participation if approached. It was felt that if the

GP was seen to be in agreement with the research, it might encourage greater participation. This was not only to be included in the postal recruitment, but also handed out to patients with families at the surgery and displayed on the walls, making the research more public.

- Those respondents who had not replied to the initial letter were to be followed up by a research health visitor who had been recruited to the study, checking addresses with practice staff and telephoning if their number was in the directory, or using 'doorstep' recruitment. While telephone numbers were generally available at the surgery, it was felt to be important to respect rights to privacy if randomly selected families had an ex-directory telephone number.

It was also decided to reduce the number of interviews from 100 to 50, selecting 30 families with preschool children and 20 with children aged 6–18. These strategies were implemented, but recruitment continued to be slow.

Table 5.2 provides an accumulative overview of the recruitment situation in May 1995, after a total of 101 people had been contacted.

Table 5.2 Accumulated recruitment summary 6 months after commencement (total contact = 101)

Method	Interviewed	Refused	Unable to contact	Moved	Response rate %
By letter	27	11	16	3	26.7
Face-to-face or telephone	3	0	20	11	29.5
Total	40	11	36	14	–

As the response rate was slightly higher for the face-to-face contacts with potential respondents who were unable to respond to the initial letter, it was decided that the remaining families would be approached personally. Data collection was completed a year after commencement.

Recruiting people for the interview phase of the research was challenging, and reasons for the difficulties experienced were not clearly established. However, several 'difficult to contact' families came from areas where disadvantage and low income predominated. It was hypothesised that participation might have been a low priority for these families, and there might have been some suspicious reluctance to be associated with 'officialdom'. This was felt to be evident in some cases where appointments had been agreed beforehand and verified immediately prior to the arranged time but the researcher was unable to gain access on arrival.

Views expressed by Thomas (1987) parallel these hypotheses. Thomas concluded that although women may agree to participate, this may indicate not their true willingness but instead their deference to authority figures. Thomas states that vulnerable families do not often value research as they have more pressing priorities. Demi and Warren (1995) add to the debate by suggesting that some families may be conducting illegal activities, such as drug use or benefit fraud, to cope with life on a low income and therefore do not take part because of a fear of exposure. Coupled with this, and although persuading some, the inclusion of a written endorsement by the GP might have acted as a further deterrent to participation, especially if relationships with or experience of health care professionals had not been optimal. Foster and Mayall (1990) suggest that this is also more likely to happen among low-income families. In addition, mobility rates among the practice population were high, and new addresses were often not presented to the practice staff until some time after the move. It was clear that the method of sample selection was becoming less 'random' and more one of 'convenience' because of the poor response rate and the difficulties experienced with contact.

It was also becoming evident that the interview data were not including the health experiences and needs of working parents, so a further recruitment plan was developed. Telephone contact was attempted during the evening to recruit families who were listed in the directory; most, however, were ex-directory or without a telephone. Two families with working parents were contacted via this method but were understandably unwilling to allow any intrusion on their valuable free time during the evenings or at weekends. In order to represent their health situation, the questionnaire that formed part of the interview schedule was modified and sent with a covering letter to 28 families in which both parents were either known or thought to be working. Selection was guided by previously contacted families who had been reluctant to participate because of working commitments. After 2 months, seven questionnaires had been returned, only three of which represented families in which both parents worked. This sample was deemed not sufficiently representative and was therefore not analysed. These examples provide additional evidence of the difficulties involved in recruitment.

Analysis

The statistical package MINITAB was used to provide descriptive and comparative information about the quantitative data collected from clients at the start of each interview. With respect to the qualitative data, a content analysis approach was used (Field and Morse, 1985). Each transcript was read in detail, and themes within the data were linked to the previously identified themes of mortality and morbidity, mental health, socioeconomic status, situation on council estates, and young people, in keeping with the pattern-matching method (Yin, 1994). As stated, the idea was to give some examples of the lived experiences of people that would perhaps provide some explanation for the seemingly poorer health outcomes indicated in the profile of people in certain areas of the town. It was appreciated, however, that concentrating overly on themes determined by profile information had the potential to miss other relevant perspectives from the interviews. In addition to this approach, therefore, further analysis was undertaken that adopted the 'salutogenic' perspective outlined earlier, looking at resources for health and coping strategies. These data used a different analytical framework and will be elaborated upon in the appropriate section below.

Results of quantitative data

The total number of respondents was 50. Most were aged between 31 and 40 years ($n = 22$), married ($n = 33$), living in households in which at least one partner was employed ($n = 35$), owned their own property ($n = 31$) and had an average of two children ($n = 35$). This latter figure rose to 3.2 in families within the manual classes and those respondents classed as 'other', which is comparable to Graham's (1984) findings, demonstrating the links between low income and family size. About a third of the sample lived in social housing ($n = 18$), and a quarter of respondents lived in households in which one partner was registered as unemployed. More than a third of respondents were from the manual classes ($n = 19$) (Registrar General's occupational classifications), and over a third again were classified as 'other' ($n = 17$), meaning in this instance single parents or unemployed. These figures are comparable to the wider demographic information obtained in the 1991 census, but unemployment within the sample was higher than local figures during 1995 (11 per cent). In general, the high levels of deprivation engendered by socio-economic status and housing that had been revealed by the wider profile were reflected in the sample. Psychological measures indicated that most people interviewed had high self-esteem, with only 8 women having low self-esteem according to the self-esteem inventory, and 2 women with high postnatal depression scores according to the Edinburgh Postnatal Depression Score.

A comparison of some of the variables with self-esteem showed that those with high self-esteem tended to be married, enjoying a good relationship with their partners and living in an owned house, at least one partner being employed. In contrast, those respondents with low self-esteem were more likely to be single or have unemployed partners, live in social housing, have a higher number of children, have less contact with family and friends over an average fortnight and perceive the health of their family to be fair or poor. In particular, most of these respondents considered their upbringing, childhood and family pressure to be currently having a bad effect upon their health. These features recur with comparison according to status, social class and housing, distinct contrasts and health experiences being apparent between married and single respondents, those owning their own property and those in social housing, those working and the unemployed, and those in the non-manual compared with the manual classes.

Results of qualitative data

The qualitative data provided a wealth of information describing the impact of social circumstances and life experiences upon the health of the respondents. The following are a selection of quotes from respondents, with their derivation code. These quotes are matched with other health and social research where appropriate to establish their relevance as indicators of need and to strengthen the emerging case description.

Making links with mortality and morbidity

The accessibility of services is highly instrumental in enabling the achievement of optimal health (Pearson *et al.*, 1993; Phillips *et al.*, 1994), yet many respondents found this to be lacking:

> the fact that they moved the hospital out of town is ridiculous... people living on this estate just can't afford to get there. (SA38:1)

As with Graham's (1987) research, several respondents highlighted the positive impact of indulging in 'unhealthy habits' regardless of the knowledge of their long-term effects:

> it helps me to cope, especially through stressful times... the urge for a cigarette overwhelms the feelings for your health. (SA43:24)

The following comment is typical of the impact and consequences of long-term unemployment:

> I'm stressed out... I did get a lot of pains in my chest, a bit worrying. (unemployed father, SA46:40)

Moser's (1986) study revealed that the death rates of unemployed men and their partners were 20 per cent higher than average death rates. He concluded that the deprivation associated with unemployment was detrimental to physical and mental health of all family members.

It sometimes seemed that food was an expensive option for some families; this again parallels comments found in research undertaken by Graham (1984):

> I've had big bills that I've had to pay back... which really leaves nothing for food at the end of the week. (SA28:5)

Cole-Hamilton and Lang's (1986) study clearly indicated the financial cost of a healthy diet for low-income families, who tend to eat less fruit and vegetables and generally have less choice with respect to healthy items.

Making links with mental health

Many of the respondents articulated the lack of control felt by having limited options:

> you just don't have the choice... you're in a certain position that you have to accept the standards that people consider are OK for you. (PS13:3)

Gilbert (1992) highlights the links between mental illness and powerlessness, indicating in particular the impact on self-esteem of limited everyday choice options. In addition, Pound *et al.* (1985) indicated that low income and poor housing are influential factors in the incidence of maternal depression, which has an impact upon the emotional development of children.

The rate of marital violence and breakdown was high:

> he tried to strangle me... there are times I've slept with a knife under my bed. (PS29:4)

> Our marriage at the end wasn't very nice... he totally ignored me... in fact I was on pills by the time he left, I'd just got myself in a mess, emotionally. (SA5:18)

The long-term impact of domestic violence upon the health of the family has been well documented (Pahl, 1981; Sadler, 1994; Kingston and Penhale, 1995). Evidence suggests that the disruption to children in later life with respect to their emotional well-being is particularly at issue. In addition, Rutter and Smith (1995) report that family conflict is associated with increased crime and the use of drugs among juveniles.

With respect to child abuse, there is overwhelming research indicating the immediate and long-term consequences of child abuse upon the health of the victim, as reviewed by Browne (1988) for example. Altemeier *et al.* (1986) demonstrated the links between the incidence of child abuse and families that experienced more disadvantage, greater isolation and more life stresses. The following quote illustrates the extent of the impact:

> The whole experience disrupted my teenage years. It screwed me up for years. (SA28:17)

Links with socioeconomic status

One client indicated the vulnerability of living with a low income:

> Being on benefit means we're so damn poor... you're also open to a lot of abuse... credit lines and things like that. (SA28:4)

Another highlighted the humiliation of applying for benefits:

> When she got her mobility allowance, she had to do the length of the corridor and the only way she could do it was on her hands and knees. (SA46:35)

Reports from the Child Poverty Action Group have repeatedly shown that the real value of benefits has decreased and is currently insufficient to cover the basic needs of the family (Lakhani, 1996a, 1996b, 1996c).

Although economic disadvantage is often linked with those who live in social housing, there are many with mortgages who find life equally stressful:

> we work and work... but we don't seem to get any benefit from it. I think it's not fair... why can't I be at home, like while they're little? I feel I'm missing out... I do suffer from depression a lot. (PS44:19)

and for single parents trying to forge a social life:

> there's constant frustrations, just a simple thing like going out for a coffee with a friend you have to think twice about. (PS25:9)

Graham (1994) demonstrated the higher levels of mental ill health among single parents who are more vulnerable to low income.

Links with social housing

The environmental hardship endured by those living on some of the estates was also harrowing:

> you get a gang come up at sort of 7 o' clock at night... you can't tell them to go away 'cos they'll put a brick through your window. (SA47:2)

That residents from 'bad' council estates reported poorer health and longstanding mental and physical illness was reported by Keithley *et al.* (1984). 'Bad' areas were characterised by high crime, poor environmant and low-quality amenities.

The amount of isolation as a result of the environment was also apparent:

It's awful here... it's just that you always seem to get certain people who go out of their way to be nasty. We hardly ever talk to anyone. (SA39:1)

For some children, the social impact of their situation was evident:

the seven year old, she'll be invited out by a friend... and then you invite them back here, as soon as they find out its this estate, well, they won't come. (PS2:6)

Graham (1984) has clearly documented the greater mental ill health experienced by women with children in poor housing situations as a result of isolation and increased caring responsibilities in adverse circumstances.

Links with children and young people

Several respondents provided graphic illustrations of the traumas they suffered as a child:

it's like my family was the kind of family that if you grew out of your clothes it was tough... I used to go to school with holes in my shoes. I don't think I could do what my mum and dad done to me. (PS19:7)

The impact of growing up in an uncaring environment has been recorded by Maccoby (1980) and Roberts (1996), who stated that the absence of security and warmth in the family results in low self-esteem of the child, a lower IQ, risky behaviour and a high level of aggression.

Another respondent illustrated well the manifestations of tension:

my friend has a flat in [estate] and she says... the parents, they're effing and blinding, they're screaming at their children, they're having screaming matches at one another all the time. (PS13:35)

There is an abundance of evidence in the literature that supports the seemingly poorer outcomes of those respondents in less advantaged situations. As demonstrated, this phase of the project provided a wealth of data supporting previous research and demonstrating intrinsic links between health and social circumstances, refocusing attention once more upon the plight of the underprivileged. Themes relating to housing, for example, confirmed it as a major health resource; as with Blackburn's (1991) review, housing can either help to protect individuals from physical and mental ill health or, as in this case, increase their vulnerability depending on its location, type and standard. The findings confirmed that tenure is strongly linked to household income in keeping with census data (OPCS, 1992), the majority of households in the lowest groups living in social housing, which previous studies show is also associated with structural, disrepair and overcrowding problems (Kemp, 1989). All these features have been shown to impact upon the psychological and physical health of individuals, increasing depression and stress (Gabe and Williams, 1986) and lowering their resistance to infection and disease (Brennan and Lancashire, 1978; Kogevinas, 1990), and the findings bear witness to this evidence.

Linked with housing are the wider environmental conditions that also have an effect on health and were evident in this study. Many low-income families were housed in urban housing complexes or areas on the periphery of towns, where there was collective poverty among the residents. These areas were characterised by poor access to community provision such as schools, playgroups and nurseries, recreational and social facilities, as well as a lack of competitively priced shops selling healthy foods. Along with the poor access to health services previously identified, there are strong links to other studies, such as Phillimore *et al.*'s (1994), which associate these environmental conditions with the growing disparities between the health outcomes of low-income groups compared with those more affluent.

Resources for health

The analysis of the data had focused upon pathological factors, but it was important now to look at how people coped in adversity to counteract this negative orientation.

Analytical framework

Theories derived from the two studies that were influential in the construction of the interview schedule were also used to develop a framework to guide the analysis of the data. First, Antonovsky's (1987) salutogenic notion of a 'sense of coherence' was used, being the extent to which people's coping and life management mechanisms can maintain them in a state of positive health. Antonovsky describes the three central components of a sense of coherence as comprehensibility, manageability and meaningfulness:

- *Comprehensibility* refers to the extent to which one perceives the stimuli one encounters, from either the internal or the external environment, as making sense and as information that is ordered, consistent and clear.
- *Manageability* refers to the extent to which one perceives that resources are available to deal with the stimuli. This may refer to resources that are under direct individual control or are accessible from family, friends or the community
- *Meaningfulness* refers to the ability to be a participant in the processes shaping one's destiny, which has the effect of enabling people to 'make sense' of events in the emotional as well as the cognitive sense.

Second, the idea of 'resources for health' developed by Cowley (1995) in her grounded theory study of health visiting was also incorporated into the analytical framework. This study looked at health as a continuous and fluctuating process, whereby people move along a continuum of illness and well-being. Transitional stages were of particular interest in this analysis with respect to identifying what factors or triggers move people from one state to the other, and what internal or external resources they draw upon that allow them to move from a negative to a positive health state. Cowley's (1995) 'health-as-process' theories were developed with health visitors, and this study provided the opportunity to test their relevance and applicability to the lay population.

Results

Interviews that had revealed particularly traumatic or frequent life events were purposefully selected for analysis using the theories outlined in order to maximise the potential for the identification of coping mechanisms and the utilisation of resources for health, and are reported fully elsewhere (Cowley and Billings, 1997). This section will provide an overview of some of the main themes using quotations and compare their significance with other health and social research.

Social support was extremely important to all respondents for a number of reasons. It provided practical resources from friends, parents or significant others, for example in paying bills, providing clothes and shoes or minding a child. Emotional support helped to reduce anger and family pressure, and the load was lightened by sharing it with someone:

> when he appeared I used to let it all out... it released a lot of my anger... it was nice... I relied on him. (PS19:36)

> I used to save up my 50ps to be able to phone her – then everything was OK again. (PS36:26)

Just knowing someone was there was sometimes sufficient.

There was evidence to suggest that rural communities were more supportive, acting collectively to help a bereaved mother and in a 'policing' fashion to discover truantees:

> people will come and tell you when your child is doing something wrong. (SA37:2)

In addition, meeting new friends acted as a powerful resource for recovery, with implications for support groups.

There are many studies that highlight the positive benefits of social support (Holahan and Moos, 1985; Oakley, 1988; Callagan and Morrissey, 1993; Whelan, 1993). Broadhead *et al.* (1983), for example, have espoused the 'buffer theory': being able to turn to people for support mitigates the effects of misfortunes and attenuates the link between adversity and the development of a psychiatric disorder.

Motherhood also acted as a powerful resource, not only giving qualities of confidence, and maturity, but also providing a focus for love in sometimes hostile environments. For some families, it appeared to furnish a means of carrying on, a trigger to do something about a situation, for example depression or hardship:

> I wasn't prepared for the love; the enjoyment, closeness and satisfaction of breastfeeding put everything else out of my mind. (PS36:7)

This view is paralleled in research undertaken by Mayall and Foster (1989) whose sample of mothers consistently expressed the positive features of childrearing, often in the face of disadvantage.

Use of the health services featured highly. Respondents spoke of their understanding and accessible GP, as illustrated by one mother whose child was a newly diagnosed asthmatic:

> he really looked after us during the worst of it, you know, and gave me lots of encouragement. I mean all those inhalers and stuff were a nightmare at first... he made me feel that I could cope with it all... and I did. (PS27)

Controversially, the use of accident and emergency services was often quoted as an important resource, particularly out of normal hours when access to more traditional health care services was more difficult.

It was, however, evident how much the respondents valued their health visitor and the home visiting service they provided, even those who were no longer in receipt of the services. Many respondents spoke warmly of the personal and therapeutic relationships they experienced with their health visitors. The following quotes are typical of the many received:

> she's more like a friend. She always listens to my moans and groans, never rushes me and I just get the feeling that she cares about me. She makes me feel a whole lot better. (PS45:19)

Such perceptions link with Cowley's (1995) notion of the health visitor as a 'resource for health'. Respondents no longer in receipt of the services also remembered their encounters with the profession, appreciating its continuity and abililty to help and support:

> 'cause I had her from the time I had my first baby until I had the twins... so that was 15 years I had her... she's one of these people, she just comes in and you think, oh it's all right, she's arrived, all my problems solved, ha ha. And she'd say to the baby, 'Oh, you're playing up again are you? I'll soon sort you out' and she used to. (SA6)

> I didn't find it intrusive, I found it incredibly helpful... she actually taught me from the beginning 'Don't worry'. I think it's the best advice I've ever had. (SA31)

Home visiting has been at the core of health visiting practice since the service was instituted in the middle of the nineteenth century, and these comments bear witness to the value placed upon it by mothers. Although undisputed measures of its effectiveness remain elusive in this country, studies in North America have demonstrated that problems in pregnancy and infancy experienced by poor unmarried teenage mothers can be alleviated by intensive home visiting programmes from appropriately trained nurses (Olds *et al.*, 1986). Follow-up studies also revealed that the number of children's injuries detected in these families was reduced for up to 2 years after the programme ended (Olds *et al.*, 1994).

Discussion

This discussion will provide a critical overview of the methodological frameworks used and their ability adequately to represent the interview data, as well as considering the extent to which the consumer perspective of need was influential in the subsequent purchasing of service provision.

With reference first to the thematic pattern-matching technique (Yin, 1994), it appeared in general to provide a relevant and meaningful framework within which to classify and order both the quantitative and the qualitative data obtained from the interviews. Some difficulties had been encountered with the phase 1 analysis of profile data relating to its complicated and time-consuming nature in the absence of information technology (Billings, 1995). However, having identified the major themes in this first phase, the qualitative analysis was able to capitalise upon the predetermined categories to order and aggregate the wide range of perceptions and views. The final case description placed the spotlight firmly upon the needs of vulnerable groups in the area.

There are some aspects of this outcome that need to be addressed. First, as discussed, the difficulties with recruitment appeared to dilute the randomness of selection, rendering it more one of convenience that had the potential to impact upon representativeness. Evidence from other previously cited studies with vulnerable families (Thomas, 1987; Demi and Warren, 1995) suggests that as access to those with the greatest need is more difficult, these respondents are in general poorly represented. However, demographic results from this research indicated a favourable comparison with the wider picture in the area, so it was felt that the study sample had captured enough disadvantaged families to render the outcome sufficiently valid.

Second, without doubt, the patterns were dominated by the health needs of the disadvantaged. While this can be partially explained, as previously discussed, by the over-reliance in phase 1 on epidemiologically related data, the health and social research appeared to support this outcome. The dependence on previous studies to justify the focus on marginalised groups can, however, have undesirable consequences. Popay *et al.* (1983), for example, state that some theories have the ability to stereotype and betray a negative orientation towards disadvantaged families or individuals. Reports on single parents such as Burghes' (1994) are implicitly condemning and can do much to reinforce popular attitudes towards them. Popay *et al.* (1983) stress that such evidence must be treated with caution. Furthermore, this method may result in a lack of recognition of the needs of the less disadvantaged sections of society. A study by Backett (1990) has highlighted significant health needs among the middle classes that are often overlooked in health needs assessments.

Despite these considerations, there is a considerable body of literature that is comparable with the findings of this study as demonstrated, and other studies concur with the notion that vulnerable groups should be specifically targeted. Reeves *et al.* (1994), for example, discovered that families headed by lone parents in the Trent area were subject to greater socioeconomic disadvantage, were younger, smoked more and suffered more relationship and housing-related stress than other family types. The authors emphasised the need to develop local health policies geared towards reversing this trend.

With reference now to the analysis of 'resources for health', the framework developed from Antonovsky's (1987) and Cowley's (1995) research provided an interesting and inter-relating way of interpreting the interview data using a salu-togenic framework. Concepts within the sense of coherence model were easier to identify following specific trauma or grief in the past, or illness of several years duration. Antonovsky's original research from which the concepts were extrapolated was concerned with Holocaust survivors years after the event. It could therefore be hypothesised that managing, comprehending and generating meaning from traumatic life events can only be understood and clearly artic-ulated following a certain time period or when the situa-tion is less intense, when reflection can perhaps take place.

The role of resources to manage this development is vital and is readily acknowledged by Antonovsky (1987). A sense of coherence and consequent ability to cope is there-fore difficult to achieve without the necessary resources. The health-as-process model (Cowley, 1995) has demon-strated the valuable link by providing a salutogenic expla-nation of how resources for health are accumulated and used to counteract the effects of critical or negative life events that may adversely affect health at individual and family levels. This method of analysis has highlighted that although a person may make sense of and recognise a negative life event, without the availability of resources or wherewithall to use them, the situation will not resolve itself positively. All the examples provided have indicated how these resources are used to maintain positive health processes and avoid negative ones, and that this transition is dependent upon recognising and establishing their availability and using them.

Given this review of the methodological approach used, the extent to which the interview data were instrumental in determining the health service provision to vulnerable families must be considered. While the profile data built upon previous research in the area to enlarge on the extent of deprivation (Cowley, 1991), the consumer perceptions and health experiences added considerable profundity and meaning to the case description, emphasising the impact of poverty. The ability of this approach to draw upon the analytical themes, unifying the data into focused specifications for practice, was realised in the form of two new posts.

First, it became clear to the purchasers that if any innovation in practice was to be introduced, it should not be at the expense of home visiting, which was acknowledged to be a valuable resource for families. In response to the clear evidence of the unmet needs of families with school-age children, the post of health visitor for school-age children was created and funded by a consortium of GP fundholders.

Second, it was by supporting the overall methodological potential in needs identification that the public health approach to service delivery was advocated. Its ability to develop programmes directed at groups in specific areas within the practice population was felt to be appropriate, localising and operationalising the broadly defined need, such as that concerning family conflict and isolation, that had been highlighted within the interview data. A community development health worker was recruited to work in one of the identified areas. Community-based initiatives have long been associated with redressing inequalities in health and enabling disadvantaged groups to influence decisions affecting their health and lives (Farrant, 1991). A further strength is their ability to incorporate the salutogenic perspective by mobilising group and community resources, for example increasing the availability of support, transport and information (Talbot, 1998).

Conclusion

Using phases of a larger project, this chapter has provided a critical account of the development of a methodology to address issues of data aggregation, representativeness and service provision with respect to consumer perceptions of need. It must be stated, however, that while this approach to data analysis can be viewed as having potential, only an evaluation of the new service provision will reveal the true extent to which the ultimately normative operationalisation of felt and expressed need in the form of the new posts is 'tokenism'. From the respondents' viewpoint, the ability of these posts to meet their needs has not been ascertained.

It is also clear that further investigation is needed to validate this method as, without additional frameworks specifically to investigate positive 'salutogenic' health states, there will be an inherent bias and valuable data for planning services will be lost. It must be remembered that the analysis of 'resources for health' was largely instrumental in revealing a specific service intervention in response to a clearly articulated need. Further to this, there will be the need to devise ways of marrying what was an intensely analytical process with practical use. If additional research demonstrates this analytical framework to be effective, further local networking will be necessary to seek out interested parties who may have the appropriate resources in place.

KEY POINTS

■ Government policy increasingly places great emphasis on seeking consumer views to inform health service planning, but there is limited guidance about how this should be achieved. There have been repeated criticisms about 'tokenism' and a lack of real influence for service users.

■ An interview survey is a potentially robust and acceptable method of identifying health needs, but achieving a sufficiently high response rate to ensure that the full range of views is represented may be problematic, especially in areas of deprivation.

KEY POINTS (cont'd)

■ Analysing data using a thematic pattern-matching approach makes it possible to set the results in the context of local statistical and epidemiological information, which is useful for informing service provision. Literature that supports or refutes the results can be integrated at this point, which increases the relevance and robustness of data identified from a small sample.

■ Lay reports about how people manage and develop their own health demonstrates their creativity and versatility in the face of adversity. Focusing solely upon 'problems' obscures this ability; analysing the data with a specific focus on positive aspects of health allows it to be revealed.

References

Altemeier R., O'Connor S., Sherrock K.B. and Tucker E. (1986) Outcome of abuse during childhood among pregnant low income women. *Child Abuse and Neglect* **10**: 319–30.

Antonovsky A. (1987) *Unravelling the Mystery of Health: How People Manage Stress and Stay Well.* San Francisco: Jossey Bass.

Backett K. (1990) Image and reality: health enhancing behaviours in middle class families. *Health Education Journal* **49**(2): 61–3.

Billings J. (1995) Investigating the Potential of Profiling in Needs Assessment and Contracting. Unpublished MSc Thesis, London: King's College, London.

Billings J. (1996) Investigating the process of community profile compilation. *Nursing Times Research* **1**(4): 270–82.

Billings J. and Cowley S. (1995) Approaches to community needs assessment: a literature review. *Journal of Advanced Nursing* **22**: 721–30.

Blackburn C. (1991) *Poverty and Health: Working with Families.* Milton Keynes: Open University Press.

Bowling A. (1992) *Local Voices in Purchasing Healthcare: An Exploratory Exercise in Public Consultation on Priority Setting.* London: Needs Assessment Unit, St Bartholomew's Hospital Medical College.

Brennan M. and Lancashire R. (1978) Association of childhood mortality with housing status and inemployment. *Journal of Epidemiology and Child Health* **32**: 28–33.

Broadhead W.E., Kaplan B.H., James S.A. and Wagner E.H. (1983) The epidemiological evidence for the relationship between social support and health. *American Journal of Epidemiology* **117**: 521–37.

Browne K. (1988) The nature of child abuse and neglect: an overview. In Browne K., Davis C. and Straton P. (eds) *Early Prediction and Prevention of Child Abuse.* Chichester: John Wiley & Sons.

Burghes L. (1994) What happens to the children of single parent families? *British Medical Journal* **308**: 1114–15.

Callagan P. and Morrissey J. (1993) Social support and health: a review. *Journal of Advanced Nursing* **18**: 203–10.

Cole-Hamilton J. and Lang T. (1986) *Tightening Belts: A Report on the Impact of Poverty on Food.* London: London Food Commission.

Cooper L., Coote A., Davies A. and Jackson C. (1995) *Voices Off. Tackling the Democratic Deficit in Health.* London: Institute for Public Policy Research.

Cowley S. (1991) Survey of Health Visiting Needs in one Practice. Consultancy Report. Hastings: Roebuck Surgery.

Cowley S. (1995) Health as process: a health visiting perspective. *Journal of Advanced Nursing* **22(3)**: 433–41.

Cowley S. and Billings J.R. (1997) The Family Health Needs Project. Final Report. London: Primary Healthcare Development Fund, King's College, London.

Cox A.D., Sagovsky R. and Cox J.L. (1987) Detection of postnatal depression: development of the ten-item Edinburgh postnatal depression scale. *British Journal of Psychiatry* **150**: 782–6.

Demi A.S. and Warren N.A. (1995) Issues in conducting research with vulnerable families. *Western Journal of Nursing Research* **17(2)**: 188–202.

Department of Health (DoH) (1989) *Working for Patients.* London: Stationery Office.

Department of Health (DoH) (1993) *Implementing Community Care: Population Needs Assessment, Good Practice Guide.* London: Stationery Office.

Department of Health (DoH) (1997) *The New NHS: Modern, Dependable.* London: Stationery Office.

Doyal L. (1983) Women's health and the sexual division of labour. *Crital Social Policy* **7**: 21–33.

Farrant W. (1991) Addressing the contradictions: health promotion and community health action in the UK. *International Journal of Health Services* **21(3)**: 423–39.

Field P. and Morse J. (1985) *Nursing Research: The Application of Qualitative Approaches.* London: Croom Helm.

Fontana A. and Frey J. (1994) Interviewing: the art of science. In Denzin N.K. and Lincoln Y.S. (eds) *Handbook of Qualitative Research.* California: Sage.

Foster M. and Mayall B. (1990) Health visitors as educators. *Journal of Advanced Nursing* **15**: 286–92.

Gabe J. and Williams P. (1986) Is space bad for your health? The relationship between crowding in the home and emotional distress in women. *Sociology of Health and Illness* **8**(4): 351–71.

Gilbert P. (1992) *Depression: The Evolution of Powerlessness.* Hove: Lawrence Erlbaum.

Goodwin S. (1994) Purchasing effective care for parents and young children. *Health Visitor* **67**(4): 127–9.

Graham H. (1984) *Women, Health and the Family.* Guilford: Wheatsheaf.

Graham H. (1987) Women's smoking and family health. *Social Science and Medicine* **25**(1): 47–56.

Graham H. (1994) The changing financial circumstances of households with children. *Children and Society* **8**(2): 98–113.

Holahan C. and Moos R. (1985) Life stress and health: personality, coping and family support in stress resistance. *Journal of Personality and Social Psychology* **49**: 739–47.

Jarman B. (1984) Underprivileged areas: validation and distribution of scores. *British Medical Journal* **289**: 1587–92.

Keithley J., Byrne D., Harrison S. and McCarthy P. (1984) Health and housing conditions in the public sector housing estates. *Public Health* **98**: 344–53.

Kemp P. (1989) The housing question. In Herbert D. and Smith D. (eds) *Social Problems and the City.* New York. Oxford University Press.

Kingston P. and Penhale B. (eds) (1995) *Family Violence and the Caring Professions.* London: Macmillan.

Kogevinas E. (1990) *1971–1983 England and Wales: Longitudinal Study. Sociodemographic Differences in Cancer Survival.* London: Stationery Office.

Lakhani B. (1996a) Welfare farewell. *Health Visitor* **69**(1): 36.

Lakhani B. (1996b) Arguing for maternity expenses. *Health Visitor* **69**(3): 112.

Lakhani B. (1996c) Desperately seeking income. *Health Visitor* **69**(5): 195.

Maccoby E.E. (1080) *Social Development: Psychological Growth and the Parent–Child Relationship.* New York: Harcourt Brace Jovanovich.

Mayall B. and Foster M.C. (1989) *Child Health Care.* London: Heinemann.

Moser K.A. (1986) *Unemployment and Mortality 1981–83. Follow-up of the 1981 Longitudinal Study Census Sample.* Working Paper 43. London: Social Statistics Research Unit, City University.

NHS Management Executive (NHSME) (1991) *Moving Forward: Needs Assessment and Contracts.* London: NHSME.

NHS Management Executive (NHSME) (1992) *Local Voices. The Views of Local People in Purchasing for Health.* London: Stationery Office.

NHS Executive (NHSE) (1995) *Priorities and Planning Guidance for the NHS: 1996/97.* London: Stationery Office.

Oakley A. (1988) Is social support good for the health of mothers and babies? *Journal of Reproductive and Infant Psychology* 6: 3–21.

Office of Population Censuses and Surveys (OPCS) (1992) *1991 Census Survey.* London: Stationery Office.

Olds D.L., Henderson C.R. and Kitzman H. (1994) Does pre-natal and infancy home visitation have an enduring effect on the qualities of parental care giving and child health at 25 to 50 months of life? *Pediatrics* 93: 89–98.

Olds D.L., Henderson C.R., Chamberlain R. and Tatelbaum R. (1986) Preventing child abuse and neglect: a randomised trial of home visitation. *Pediatrics* 78: 65–78.

Pahl J. (ed.) (1981) *Private Violence and Public Policy.* London: Routledge & Kegan Paul.

Pearson M., Dawson C., Moore H. and Spence S. (1993) Health on borrowed time? Prioritising and meeting needs in low income families. *Health and Social Care in the Community* 1(1): 45–59.

Peckham S. and Spanton J. (1994) Community development approaches to health needs assessment. *Health Visitor* 67(4): 124–5.

Phillimore P., Beattie A. and Townsend P. (1994) Widening inequality of health in northern England, 1981–91. *British Medical Journal* 308: 1125–8.

Phillips C., Palfrey C. and Thomas P. (1994) *Evaluating Health and Social Care.* Basingstoke: Macmillan.

Popay J., Rimmer L. and Rossiter C. (1983) *One Parent Families: Parents, Children and Public Policy. Study Commission on the Family.* Occasional Paper No. 12. London: Study Commission on the Family.

Pound A., Cox A., Puckering C. and Mills M. (1985) The impact of maternal depression on young children. In Stevenson J. (ed.) *Recent Research in Developmental Psychology.* London: Sage.

Reeves J., Kendrick D., Denman S. and Roberts H. (1994) Lone mothers: their health and lifestyle. *Health Education Journal* 53: 291–9.

Richards J. (1991) Consumer-oriented planning. In *Social Services Inspectorate Community Care Plans – the First Steps.* London: Stationery Office.

Roberts I. (1996) Family support and the health of children. *Children and Society* 10: 217–24.

Rodgers J. (1994) Power to the people. *Health Service Journal* 104(5395): 28–9.

Rosenberg M. (1965) *Society and the Adolescent Self-Image.* Princeton, NJ: Princeton University Press.

Rutter M. and Smith D. (1995) *Psychosocial Disorders in Young People: Time, Trends and their Causes.* Chichester: John Wiley & Sons.

Sadler C. (1994) Domestic violence: hidden from help. *Health Visitor* **67**(6): 185–6.

Stalker K. (1993) The best laid plans... gang aft agley? Assessing population needs in Scotland. *Health and Social Care* **2**: 1–9.

Talbot S. (1998) A community approach to health. In *Poverty and Public Health: Finally on the Agenda.* London: CPHVA.

Thomas R.B. (1987) Methodological issues and problems in family healthcare research. *Journal of Marriage and the Family* **49**: 65–70.

Whelan C.T. (1993) The role of social support in mediating the psychological consequences of economic stress. *Sociology of Health and Illness* **15**(1): 87–101.

Yin R.K. (1994) *Case Study Research: Design and Methods.* Newbury Park, CA: Sage.

6

Client Perceptions of the Health Visiting Service

Ina Machen

This chapter presents a research project that examined whether health visiting, which emerged at the end of the nineteenth century, is relevant to contemporary first-time mothers. Although previous studies have explored clients' perceptions of health visiting, the fundamental question of whether or not the provision of such a service was needed or wanted by mothers of today had not been addressed. In this descriptive qualitative study, 20 first-time mothers from a small cluster sample were interviewed in their own homes. The findings indicate that a client-centred health visiting service is highly relevant to the needs of contemporary first-time mothers and can be a service that is greatly valued.

Background

The policy to establish a health visiting service in the UK, with the aim of promoting the health of babies and young children by the education and support of mothers, evolved during the latter part of the nineteenth century and the early twentieth century (Dingwall, 1977; Prochaska, 1980; Robinson, 1982; Dwork, 1987; Dingwall *et al.*, 1988). Although provision was at first localised and uneven, the Maternity and Child Welfare Act of 1918 provided the necessary legislation to enable a national health visiting service to develop. This was very much supported by working-class women, who campaigned for maternal and child welfare services (Llewelyn-Davies, 1978).

Today, despite many far-reaching social, medical, economic and political changes in society, and therefore in the lives of women (Lewis, 1984, 1992), the policy continues to be implemented. This, then, raises the question of how far such a service developed in a very different social and political context is relevant to women today. This was the fundamental question to be addressed by the research since it was considered important that health visitors, searching for health needs, understand whether the core service (support for new mothers) is indeed wanted or valued by today's clients. With such an understanding, the search for health needs could be more effectively pursued. Unfortunately, the needs and perceptions of fathers are beyond the scope of this research project.

Review of the literature

There are numerous studies of consumer perceptions of health visiting, such as those of Field *et al.* (1982), Clark (1984), Simms and Smith (1984), Sefi (1985), McIntosh (1986), Cubbon (1987), Weatherley (1988), Mayall and Foster (1989) and Cameron (1990), but these do not directly address the question of the contemporary relevance of the service to clients. Nevertheless, these studies do expose certain issues of concern that are pertinent to the present discussion.

First, the literature revealed a wide range in the level of consumer satisfaction in relation to home visits and clinics. For example, Weatherley's (1988) survey of a 25 per cent sample of families on one health visitor's caseload found high levels of satisfaction in relation to the frequency of home visits. However, in McIntosh's study of first-time working-class mothers, only 3 out of 59 (5 per cent) spoke in favour of home visits, while 21 out of 59 (36 per cent) expressed a dislike of the health visitor calling at home. With regard to clinics, Field *et al.* (1982) reported that many mothers found the clinics busy and unfriendly places that lacked privacy. In contrast, Cubbon (1987) found high levels of satisfaction with clinics, especially in relation to the re-assurance that parents received about their child's progress.

Second, in terms of the role and function of health visi-tors, several studies highlighted consumer confusion over the role of the health visitor, especially in relation to the support and surveillance aspects of the service. For example, Graham (1979), who provided one of the earlier surveys, identified the conflict in the health visiting role between offering support and at the same time policing aspects of the mother's work. Graham found that this seemed to arouse feelings of inadequacy and embarrass-ment in working-class and first-time mothers.

Orr's (1980) study of the views of 68 Northern Ireland mothers also identified this dichotomy and found that participants saw health visiting as either relationship centred or as problem centred. Robinson (1982), Sefi (1985), Mayall and Grossmith (1985) and McIntosh (1986) similarly found evidence of this dual approach in health visiting, which created uncertainties concerning the health visitors' appropriate role and function. Gott (1991, 1992), in a later study, found that participants mainly believed that the health visitor checked to see that babies were progressing normally, while the preventive aspect of her role went largely unrecognised. The level of ignorance and misconception regarding the health visitor's role as well as the conflicts inherent within it, which these studies have exposed, have important implications for women's percep-tions of the health visiting service as a potential resource and their effective use of it.

A third issue highlighted by the literature was the evidence that women may be undermined by health visiting interventions, especially through the authoritarian 'top-down' health education approach that health visitors some-times adopt (Sefi, 1985; McIntosh, 1986; Billingham, 1989; Foster and Mayall, 1990). Unsolicited advice appeared to be less acceptable than advice specifically requested as participants preferred health visitors to be responsive to *their* needs and to engage in discussion relevant to *their* concerns. The authoritarian approach, therefore, was revealed by these studies to be counterproductive.

Thus, the research highlighted that there are aspects of the service that may actually have a negative outcome. That some women felt undermined, or thought that the health visitor's role was primarily that of inspector, was a serious charge demanding closer scrutiny. This research project sought to explore these issues as part of its broader objective of gaining an understanding of the contemporary relevance of the service. This seems particularly important at a time of radical change within the British NHS as a result of the NHS and Community Care Act 1990 (DoH, 1990), the impetus for a primary care-led NHS through the establishment of Primary Care Groups (PCGs) (DoH, 1997), the recent government consultation document, 'Supporting Families' (Home Office, 1998) and the increasing emphasis on clinical effectiveness (DoH, 1998).

The study

The overall aim of this descriptive study was to gain information concerning women's perceptions of the relevance of the health visiting service to their needs. A total of 20 women were interviewed 4–6 months after the birth of their first baby. A further three women were interviewed for the pilot study. The researcher conducted all the interviews, which lasted between 45 and 80 minutes. Field notes were taken and parts of the interviews were audiotaped and transcribed.

Research design

Of great importance in this study was the need to use a research method that would lead to an increased understanding of the relevance of the service to the main client group – new mothers. It was thus important to hear the views and experiences of the women in their own words. Accordingly, a broadly interpretative/feminist methodology appeared to be the most appropriate (Roberts, 1981; Nielsen, 1990; Lincoln, 1992). Although the sample was small owing to limitations of time and resources, this was counterbalanced by the descriptive range, richness of data and additional understanding that qualitative research offers.

It was decided that semi-structured interviews would be conducted in the women's own homes. It was hoped that this non-threatening environment would encourage the development of a good rapport between researcher and participant. In keeping with feminist research methodology, the 'interactive' interviews would as far as possible not seek to exploit participants as 'objects of data', rejecting the assumption that maintains a strict separation between researcher and research subject (Oakley, 1981; Nielsen, 1990; Lincoln, 1992).

As it was not possible to audiotape each interview in its entirety because of time and resource constraints, field notes were taken during the initial stages. It was also thought that not recording the early part of the interview would give participants time to feel comfortable with the researcher and the interview process before recording commenced. The topic guide consisted mainly of open-ended questions that focused discussion on different aspects of the service. Ethical approval for the study was obtained, and permission was given by the chief nurse of an NHS Trust to use data from the Notification of Births register to draw up a representative cluster sample of first-time mothers. The research was discussed with the local neighbourhood manager and health visitors, who were supportive of the study.

Sample and pilot work

As it was important in this study that the perceptions of a range of first-time mothers were obtained, it was decided that, although this was a qualitative research project, a cluster sample would provide the best means of ensuring that clients from a variety of sociocultural backgrounds, including clinic non-attenders, were represented.

The sample included all women living in a small manufacturing town in the home counties of England (population approximately 27 000) whose first baby was born in a particular 2-month period in 1993. It was initially expected that the sample would be drawn from the mothers of babies born in a single month, but as this produced an insufficient number of first-time mothers, the time frame was extended to cover a 2-month period. The small cluster sample finally consisted of 22 women. The data, obtained from the birth notifications, were checked against current computerised health visiting records to ensure that all the details were accurate and that the first contact, by letter, would be appropriate, that is, that no infant deaths or serious illnesses had occurred. Although there were no such problems, three families had moved (albeit remaining within the town), and three babies had been registered under a different name, which made cross-checking data rather difficult. As is so often the case in research, the process of obtaining the sample and checking the details was far more time consuming and complex than had been anticipated.

As the sample was small, the number of variables was kept to a minimum. Therefore, only first-time mothers were selected, who, at the time of interview, had had between 4 and 6 months' experience of the health visiting service (excluding any antenatal contact), mostly in the form of home visits and clinic attendance. A cluster sample had the advantage of excluding other variables relating to differences in policy implementation between districts. The sample covered the caseloads of five different health visitors and three GP practices. The response rate was high. There were 20 participants from the total sample of 22 mothers. All the women in the sample in fact agreed to participate initially, but two withdrew at the time of data collection, one because of illness and the other because of family difficulties.

Three pilot interviews were conducted with first-time mothers in a different geographical area who had babies of approximately 4 months of age; minor amendments were subsequently made to the topic guide. The experience enabled the researcher to practise and refine interview skills.

Data collection

Initial contact by letter, which introduced the researcher and described the project, was followed up 7–10 days later by a telephone call to ascertain whether the mother would be willing to participate. If so, an interview (in her home and at her convenience) was arranged. Participants' verbal consent was obtained at the time of the interview and issues relating to ensuring confidentiality, which had been referred to in the letter, were discussed in more detail. Participants' permission was sought for field notes to be taken during interviews and for part of the interviews to be audiotaped. One participant did not wish to be audiotaped but was happy for field notes to be taken. The participants appeared to be very willing and eager to tell of their experiences and perceptions of the health visiting service.

As reflexivity is an important aspect of qualitative research (Webb, 1992), a field diary recording the context of the interview, non-verbal communication and the researcher's perceptions of the interview process was completed following each interview. It was hoped that this information would be helpful both in conducting subsequent interviews and during data analysis. As soon after each interview as possible, the field notes were read through and the tapes were transcribed. To ensure anonymity, each participant was given a code number that was used to identify her interview schedule, audiotape and entry in the field diary.

Rigour and auditability

The application of validity and reliability measures in qualitative research remains controversial (Hammersley, 1992; Webb, 1992). Various terms have been suggested to describe alternative approaches to establishing rigour in qualitative research. For example, Guba and Lincoln (1981) suggest 'auditability' as a criterion of rigour, that is, the ability of another person readily to follow the 'decision trail' used by the researcher in the study. For this to occur, the progress of events in the study must be presented so that their logic is clear (Webb, 1992). Such an approach was adopted in this study, albeit within the constraints of financial resources and time. Also, an open, reflective style was employed to enhance credibility (Hammersley and Atkinson, 1983; Webb, 1992).

To avoid bias, the first contact letter to the women in the sample did not explicitly state that the researcher was a health visitor but explained that she worked for an NHS Trust and was undertaking research.

Data analysis

The topic guide focused discussion on five aspects of the service, namely home visits, clinics, access to health visitors, advice and general aspects of the service. Probes were included to enable the discussion to delve more deeply if required. Hence, the interviews were semi-structured rather than unstructured discussions, but the questions were as far as possible open ended.

Analytical categories

At the end of the study, the interview transcripts and field notes were reviewed in order to identify topics, themes or issues contained in the open-ended responses, including the contexts in which statements were made. The data were subjected to three-stage analysis as reported by Miles and Huberman (1984): data reduction, data display and conclusion-drawing. The emergent themes and topics were subsequently categorised and analysed using the initial coding process described by Chenitz and Swanson (1986). To ensure that the data were analysed in context, transcripts and field notes were referred to at frequent intervals throughout the process so that the participants' original meaning was maintained. This method had the advantage that analytical categories were derived as far as possible from the data rather than being predetermined. Respondent validation of the categorisation process was considered but omitted, not only owing to time and resource constraints, but also because the validity of this process is questionable (Hammersley and Atkinson, 1983; Sandelowski, 1993).

Five main analytical categories emerged:

1. *Effectiveness:* the effectiveness/usefulness/influence of, and satisfaction with, the service. The underlying theme was how appropriate and how good the service was, as perceived by clients.
2. *Acceptability:* the acceptability of health visiting policy to women. The underlying theme was whether this unsolicited service was perceived as being intrusive or interfering.
3. *Users' assessment:* the participants' perceptions of the health visitor's role and function. The underlying theme was the users' understanding of what the service offered.
4. *Relevance:* the relevance/appropriateness of the policy from the mother's perspective. The underlying theme was the general 'fit' of the service with women's needs.
5. *Facilitative or controlling/directive:* the extent to which the service was perceived by mothers as controlling or empowering. The underlying theme was whether health visiting policy empowered, or undermined and controlled.

Results of the study

Demographic details

The age of the 20 participants ranged from 18 to 39 years. There were certain problems in stratifying the sample according to class, owing to the inherent problems associated with this form of classification for women (Goldthorpe, 1984; Blaxter, 1990; Davis, 1992). However, the sample was crudely divided into working-class and middle-class groupings based mainly on income and the participant's present or previous occupation, giving figures of 10 middle-class, 7 working-class, and 3 unemployed women. Interestingly, the responses did not show any pattern in relation to class. This suggested that, for these participants, the experience of motherhood transcended socioeconomic influence. With a small sample, a pattern is less likely to emerge, but Foxman *et al.* (1982) and Pearson (1991) also found that socioeconomic factors had little effect on clients' perceptions of health visiting. The vast majority of the women were British; only two participants were not born in the UK, but both had lived and worked in Britain for some years.

General aspects of the health visiting service

The data analysis was a lengthy process, and the volume of data produced by the interviews was far greater than had been anticipated. Therefore, the presentation of the findings is selective, focusing on participants' perceptions of the service overall in relation to the five analytical categories outlined above. In the selection of participant comments, an attempt has been made to communicate most economically and vividly the mothers' perceptions. The selection also attempts, where appropriate, to represent the majority view as accurately as possible.

Effectiveness

With respect to the effectiveness of the service as a whole, very high levels of satisfaction were recorded. The vast majority of participants (19) found the service, overall, to be either helpful or very helpful:

Very good – I wouldn't be without it. Brilliant! (Participant 1)

Yes, definitely very helpful – a first-class service. (Participant 10)

A great help… I needed the advice and back-up. (Participant 20)

It is also very significant that, in response to a direct question concerning the amount of contact with the service, none of the mothers wanted less. A small majority of women (11) found the amount of contact about right for their needs:

It was fine for me as it was. They were there when I needed them. (Participant 15)

It's about right. It's up to me how I want to use the service. (Participant 3)

It's just about right. You have the freedom to go [to the clinic]. (Participant 16)

A large minority (9) would have preferred more contact:

I would like to have more contact, but at home. (Participant 6)

In the early days I would have preferred more [contact]. (Participant 7)

It appeared that the service was valued and needed by the mothers, and, significantly, many expressed a preference for more contact, especially through home visits. It is important to note here that such high levels of satisfaction have not been found in other studies, although a comparison is difficult because of variations in the sampling frames and methods used. However, to help to gauge the significance of these findings, it can be noted that Clark (1984) found 70 per cent of her sample to have perceived the health visitor as being helpful, a percentage similar to that reported by Graham (1979), Orr (1980), Foxman *et al.* (1982) and Weatherley (1988). In contrast, McIntosh (1986) found that only 40 per cent of participants reported receiving any useful help or advice from their health visitor. Sherratt *et al.* (1991) found that only 27 per cent of mothers in her study gave positive comments about the service.

The high levels of satisfaction recorded in this study may in part be explained by the fact that all the participants were first time-mothers who, being new to motherhood, were more likely to need support. However, McIntosh's (1986) study was also of first-time mothers. It is perhaps more likely that the greater satisfaction is related to changes in the approach of health visitors. This issue is considered in the discussion below.

Acceptability

There is evidence that, since the beginning of the health visiting service, many families have regarded the home visit as intruding into their privacy (Davin, 1978; Robinson, 1982; Lewis, 1986; Steedman, 1986). However, in this study, nine participants commented that, while others may find the home visit unacceptable, they themselves did not find it intrusive:

> I look forward to her visits. If people do [find them intrusive] I think they have something to hide. That's my personal opinion. (Participant 10)

> I don't find the visits intrusive… How health visitors interact with clients is important. My sister said her health visitor 12 years ago seemed to inspect the house – asked to go to the loo or wash her hands to have a look around, she felt. (Participant 17)

McIntosh (1986) also found that several mothers commented that health visitors tried to inspect their homes surreptitiously. In fact, all the women in this study (20) found the visits to be acceptable and non-intrusive:

> She will phone to see what time it is convenient for me. No, it's not intrusive, I feel glad to have her visit. (Participant 21)

> I didn't find that with my health visitor. I thought it would be like that when I first heard I was to have a health visitor, but it wasn't. They seemed genuinely interested in you and in the baby's well-being, and nothing else really. (Participant 16)

> I certainly didn't find them intrusive. I found them a *great* help. (Participant 3)

This result must reflect, in part, the interpersonal skills of the health visitors involved and the fact that most home visiting is nowadays prearranged. Mothers seemed to value this:

> If they don't phone before, they could be [intrusive]. Both visits I had were arranged. (Participant 5)

Users' assessment

The literature revealed that there were misconceptions concerning the health visitor's role (Clark, 1984; McIntosh, 1986; Pearson, 1991). The women in this study, however, appeared to have a good understanding. When asked directly about the health visitor's role, the aspect most frequently highlighted was the help, advice and support *for mothers*.

> To give us help and confidence. (Participant 1)

> To look after mother and baby – but maybe more so us. (Participant 4)

> Giving advice and guidance – being there for the mother. (Participant 16)

Bearing in mind that health visitors were visiting the participants because they had children, it is interesting that the function acknowledged most frequently was not the health visitors' direct role with the child but help and support for mothers. The health visitor's role in the care and well-being of the baby was articulated, albeit less frequently.

Only a small minority of participants referred to the surveillance aspect of the health visitor's work, commenting that health visitors 'check' the suitability of the home, the care of the baby or the mother's ability to cope. That so few participants made reference to this aspect of the role contrasts with the findings of other studies. For example, Mayall and Foster (1989) found that their sample perceived the major role of the health visitor to be that of inspecting households to detect child abuse. In the research by McIntosh (1986), 56 per cent of the sample described the role of the health visitor exclusively in terms of social control.

It appears that, for many mothers in this study, the health visitor's role was mainly perceived to be that of offering help, advice, support and reassurance, as well as of caring for the well-being of the baby and mother. The following quotations highlight clearly that, although perceptions of the stereotypical policing function of the health visitor still persist, they were dispelled for many participants by the health visitors themselves:

What you hear before you have a baby is very much the social services type thing – you hear about the problems over kids who are mistreated and so on, and therefore you seem to think of them in the role of watching to make sure you are bringing up your child correctly. You think of them in a policing role, rather than a helpful role. It's not until you have the baby that you strike up a relationship with them and you realise that they actually have a very different role... generally giving you information that you can't necessarily get from elsewhere. (Participant 2)

Another participant stated:

I thought it would be inspecting me when they came round... really checking up on you. (Participant 16)

This mother went on to say that she had found the service very helpful and that she now saw the health visitor's role as giving advice and 'generally being there for the mother'. It is important to highlight at this point that the service provided by the health visitors, which was perceived very positively by the sample, had actually been viewed by many of the participants, prior to contact, in a very negative light. The health visitors had been successful in breaking down these stereotypical images of the service. This must, in no small way, reflect their professional and communication skills, and the personalities of the health visitors themselves, for, as Clark (1984) has suggested, the personal attributes of the health visitor are an important factor in consumer satisfaction with the service. Thus, in the main, the users' assessment of the health visitor's role did not reflect previous studies, which emphasised their policing function, but showed a good understanding and appreciation of their supportive and information-giving functions, although their health-promotion role was mentioned specifically by only one participant.

Relevance

Towards the end of the interview, mothers were asked whether it would matter if we did not have health visitors. All the participants (20) felt that the service was needed. Only one mother stated that, although she could manage without, other mothers in less favourable circumstances would be disadvantaged. The other participants valued the service for themselves. It was in response to this question that many women referred to the surveillance role of the health visitor as a necessary function to protect children:

> Others would have to do the job if they weren't here, such as doctors... Kids would be in danger or suffer. (Participant 11)

Several women mentioned that without the health visiting service, doctors' workloads would be greater:

> If I have any problems I'd see her [the health visitor] before I go to the doctor... I'd have to bother the doctor a lot more... Where would you get her weighed and get all the things the health visitors do? (Participant 6)

> You can talk to them without going to the doctor. They have an important role to play. It's a service we couldn't do without, and it's taken for granted. They do a lot more work than people actually see. Doctors would be a lot busier and troubled with a lot of things they needn't be. There would be a lot of less well looked after babies and children. (Participant 8)

These results stand out in sharp contrast to those of McIntosh (1986), who found that only 23 per cent of respondents felt that they personally would miss the service if it did not exist.

Facilitative or controlling/directive

A problem identified in the literature was the way in which the health visiting service was seen to undermine mothers rather than support or empower them. It was therefore important that this one issue was specifically addressed in the interviews. Only one mother felt that health visitors had underestimated her abilities as a mother; two felt that they sometimes had and two were unsure:

> She felt I knew what I was doing. I don't think so – maybe she did... A difficult question for me to answer. (Participant 8)

> It's difficult for me to say. Health visitors could be over-officious... this is down to individual personality. (Participant 18)

In answer to the question, 'Do you feel that the health visitor values the skills and knowledge you have as a mother, or do you feel that she underestimates your abilities?', 15 mothers felt that their abilities had not been underestimated, and the non-directive approach was praised by several. The first quotation below draws out the contrast between this approach and the more authoritarian style criticised in other studies:

> No, they never do. They always boost your confidence... My sister-in-law was scared out of her life by her health visitor. They were like school teachers then. (Participant 1)

> Generally I know my health visitor made me feel I was capable and could handle the situation. She waited for me to ask the questions, rather than saying you should do this or that. She didn't undervalue me as a mother. (Participant 3)

> No, I think the way she was talking to me was as if she just wanted to be there for a source of information, and if I had any problems. (Participant 13)

Thus, three-quarters of the mothers saw the service as facilitative rather than controlling or directive. As the above comments demonstrate, a large majority of the mothers felt empowered by their health visitors and were encouraged to use them as a resource. The health visitors were perceived as recognising and valuing the mothers' knowledge and providing the opportunity for them to seek information or help when they needed it. Again, these results were far more favourable than those of other authors, such as Sefi (1985), McIntosh (1986) and Mayall and Foster (1989). These studies all provide evidence of participants' dissatisfaction with unsolicited advice and the authoritarian approach adopted by the health visitors. Perhaps the findings presented here reflect a change in approach for health visiting since the 1980s, which emphasises the use of non-directive interpersonal skills. One of the current aims of health promotion is empowerment, and we have seen here that this facilitative approach, on the whole, provides a relevant, effective and acceptable service to mothers.

Limitations of the study

There were clearly limitations to this study. It provided only a 'snapshot' view of mothers' perceptions of the service. There is evidence from other studies (see especially Graham, 1979) that clients' satisfaction declines over time. Therefore, the favourable findings must be interpreted with caution. Also, the research focused on only one area of the health visiting service: the provision for new mothers and babies. Although this is probably the priority client group, other aspects of the service have been neglected. As Blaxter (1990) highlights, attitudes and opinions expressed in a study such as this are 'presentations' to the interviewer, and we cannot know what relationship they bear to what participants 'really' think, especially as they were only interviewed once. However, the women did appear to speak freely and frankly during the interviews.

The social class stratification of the participants was a problem, not only because of the great difficulties of assigning socioeconomic status to women, but also because of the inadequate data obtained. More detailed questions should have been asked about occupation, educational attainment and income. In addition, and most importantly, this was a small study concerning the relevance of the health visiting service to a small sample of mothers with young babies in one small town. Therefore, it does not purport to be a representative study. Nevertheless, it is hoped that the results will be useful to policy-makers, health visitors and managers.

Implications for health visiting and further research

The consumer view reported in this study was based on the opinions of a small and probably unrepresentative sample of mothers in a single area. Its contribution is in addressing the fundamental issue of the relevance of health visiting policy to contemporary mothers. The study has provided evidence that health visiting policy is highly relevant to the needs of contemporary mothers. The high levels of satisfaction revealed that, on the whole, the needs of mothers were being met in a way that they found effective and acceptable. The implication for practice, therefore, is that the facilitative approach of health visitors empowers mothers and appears to be appreciated and effective. A more authoritarian and directive approach, as the literature highlights, appears to be less acceptable. The apparent correlation between high levels of consumer satisfaction and the facilitative approach of health visitors requires further research.

Perhaps the most important implication for health visiting is that the study identifies that there continues to be a real demand for the service, so long as it is responsive and sensitive to the needs of mothers. In the light of the changes that are presently occurring within the NHS, it is evident that health visiting policy will be revised and rationalised. It would be regrettable to see a service eroded that seems to be providing the kind of advice and support for which women had campaigned at the beginning of the twentieth century (Llewellyn-Davies, 1978) and which was so valued by the women in this study.

Another implication for health visiting is that, prior to any contact with the service, many participants thought that the visits would be intrusive and 'inspecting' in character. If the emphasis has shifted away from this approach, perhaps the service needs some positive marketing to improve its image. It has a low profile in the media generally and tends to be mentioned only in relation to cases of child abuse. As previously stated, misconceptions about the service have important implications for women's perceptions of health visiting as a potential resource for them and their utilisation of the service. Once the participants in this study had contact with health visitors, the resource aspect of the service was recognised and valued, although the controlling function was also acknowledged. The concern of the women for *all* children in society seemed to provide the justification and acceptability for the surveillance aspect of health visiting. It is possible that the health visiting service would be less acceptable if it were targeted only at particular families. This is an area that requires further research.

More research is also required to identify the most cost-effective way to provide the support and advice that new mothers need. Skill mix and an increased role for the voluntary sector may be the way forward; however, this study has highlighted that the interpersonal skills and knowledge of health visitors were highly valued by mothers. Therefore, it is important that this level of expertise continues to be available. The major problem is clearly how to measure or assess what is *prevented* by health visiting intervention.

Many participants in this study thought that morbidity rates would be higher if health visitors were not available:

> Kids would be in danger or suffer. (Participant 2)

> There would be a lot of less well looked after babies and children. (Participant 20)

> I think that there would possibly be more mums going round the bend, and more children getting hurt or neglected. (Participant 18)

Demonstrating and assessing the health outcomes of health visiting policy remains an important and urgent challenge for health visitors.

KEY POINTS

- In-depth interviews avoid creating a hierarchical relationship between interviewer and participant and facilitate the easy flow of information – Lofland's (1971) 'guided conversation'. This enables participants to articulate their perceptions and experiences in their own words, providing rich, detailed material for qualitative analysis.

- The health visiting service's adoption of a client-centred approach is relevant to the needs of contemporary first-time mothers.

- It is important that health visitors and professional organisations continue to promote a more positive and up-to-date image of health visiting to correct misconceptions about the role that may be held by new mothers.

KEY POINTS (cont'd)

■ The acceptability of the surveillance aspect of the health visitor's role appeared to be associated with the universality of the service. This may have implications for a targeted service and requires further research.The non-directive approach of the health visitors was highly valued by participants and facilitated the development of empowering relationships. It is important that the curriculum for the education of health visitors and other primary health care nurses continues to promote the development of effective interpersonal and counselling skills.

■ Participants very much appreciated the broad knowledge base of the health visitors. Parents' access to this level of health visiting expertise may be reduced by a skill mix that involves less direct contact between parents and health visitors as aspects of the health visitors' work are increasingly delegated to junior members of the health visiting team. The implications and cost-effectiveness of such skill mix deserve further research.

Acknowledgement

I should like to thank all the women who participated in the study and the health visitors for their time and support.

References

Billingham K. (1989) 45 Cope Street. *Community Outlook* 8(1): 8–10.

Blaxter M. (1990) *Health and Lifestyle.* London: Tavistock/Routledge.

Cameron S. (1990) Clients' perception of a home visit. *Focus, Scottish Health Visitors' Association Magazine* 19: 22–3

Chenitz W.C. and Swanson J.M. (1986) *From Practice to Grounded Theory: Qualitative Research in Nursing.* Menlo Park, CA: Addison Wesley.

Clark J. (1984) Mothers' perceptions of health visiting. *Health Visitor* 57(9): 265–8.

Cubbon J. (1987) Consumer attitudes to child health clinics. *Health Visitor* 60(6): 185–6.

Davin A. (1978) Imperialism and motherhood. *History Workshop Journal* 5: 9–65.

Davis H. (1992) Social stratification in Europe. In Bailey J. (ed.) *Social Europe.* Harlow: Longman.

Department of Health (DoH) (1990) *The NHS and Community Care Act 1990.* London: HMSO.

Department of Health (DoH) (1997) *The New NHS: Modern, Dependable.* Cmnd 3809. London: Stationery Office.

Department of Health (DoH) (1998) *A First Class Service: Quality in the New NHS.* London: Stationery Office.

Dingwall R. (1977) Collectivism, regionalism and feminism: health visiting policy 1850–1975. *Journal of Social Policy* **6**(3): 291–315.

Dingwall R., Rafferty A.M. and Webster C. (1988) *An Introduction to the Social History of Nursing.* London: Routledge.

Dwork D. (1987) *War is Good for Babies and Other Young Children.* London: Tavistock.

Field S., Draper J., Kerr M. and Hare M. (1982) A consumer view of the health visiting service. *Health Visitor* **55**(6): 299–301.

Foster M.-C. and Mayall B. (1990) Health visitors as educators. *Journal of Advanced Nursing* **15**: 286–92.

Foxman R., Moss P., Bollard G. and Owen C. (1982) A consumer view of the health visitor at six weeks postpartum. *Health Visitor* **55**(6): 302–8.

Goldthorpe J. (1984) Women and class analysis: a reply to the replies. *Sociology* **18**(4): 491–9.

Gott M (1991) *North Staffordshire Quality Project.* Stoke-upon-Trent: North Staffordshire Community Trust.

Gott M. (1992) Measuring quality in community nursing. *Professional Care of Mother and Child* (Sep): 236.

Graham H. (1979) Women's attitudes to the child health services. *Health Visitor* **52**(5): 175–8.

Guba E. and Lincoln Y. (1981) *Effective Evaluation.* San Francisco: Jossey-Bass.

Hammersley M. (1992) *What's Wrong with Ethnography?* London: Routledge.

Hammersley M. and Atkinson P. (1983) *Ethnography: Principles in Practice.* London: Tavistock.

Home Office (1998) *Supporting Families: A Consultation Document.* London: Stationery Office.

Lewis J. (1984) *Women in England 1870–1950.* London: Harvester Wheatsheaf.

Lewis J. (1986) The working class wife and mother and state intervention 1870–1918. In Lewis J. (ed.) *Labour and Love.* Oxford: Basil Blackwell.

Lewis J. (1992) *Women in Britain Since 1945.* Oxford: Basil Blackwell.

Lincoln Y.S. (1992) Sympathetic connections between qualitative methods and health research. *Qualitative Health Research* **2**(4): 375–91.

Llewelyn-Davies M. (ed.) (1978) *Maternity, Letters From Working Women.* London: Virago. (First published 1915.)

Lofland J. (1971) *Analysing Social Settings.* Belmont, CA: Wadsworth.
McIntosh J. (1986) *A Consumer Perspective on the Health Visiting Service.* Glasgow: Department of Child Health and Obstetrics, University of Glasgow.
Mayall B. and Foster M.-C. (1989) *Child Health Care.* Oxford: Heinemann.
Mayall B. and Grossmith C. (1985) The health visitor and the provision of services. *Health Visitor* **58**(12): 349–52.
Miles M.B. and Huberman A.M. (1984) *Qualitative Data Analysis.* London: Sage.
Nielsen J.M. (1990) Introduction. In Nielsen J.M. (ed.) *Feminist Research Methods.* London: Westview Press.
Oakley A. (1981) Interviewing women: a contradiction in terms. In Roberts A. (ed.) *Doing Feminist Research.* London: Routledge & Kegan Paul.
Orr J. (1980) *Health Visiting in Focus.* London: RCN.
Pearson P. (1991) Clients' perceptions: the use of case studies in developing theory. *Journal of Advanced Nursing* **16**: 521–8.
Prochaska F. (1980) *Women and Philanthropy in Nineteenth Century England.* Oxford: Clarendon Press.
Roberts H. (1981) Introduction. In Roberts H. (ed.) *Doing Feminist Research.* London: Routledge & Kegan Paul.
Robinson J. (1982) *An Evaluation of Health Visiting.* London: CETHV.
Sandelowski M. (1993) Rigor or rigor mortis: the problem of rigor in qualitative research revisited. *Advances in Nursing Science* **16**(2): 1–8.
Sefi S. (1985) The First Visit: A Study of Health Visitor/Mother Verbal Interactions. Unpublished MA dissertation, Department of Sociology, University of Warwick.
Sherratt F., Johnson A. and Holmes S. (1991) Responding to parental concerns at the six-month stage. *Health Visitor* **64**(3): 84–6.
Simms M. and Smith C. (1984) Teenage mothers: some views on health visitors. *Health Visitor* **57**(9): 269–70.
Steedman C. (1986) *Landscape for a Good Woman.* London: Virago.
Weatherley D. (1988) A survey of clients' views in one health visitor's caseload. *Health Visitor* **61**(5): 137–8.
Webb C. (1992) The use of the first person in academic writing: objectivity, language, and gatekeeping. *Journal of Advanced Nursing* **17**: 747–75.

7

Researching the Health Needs of Mothers in Low-income Households

Clare Blackburn

A significant increase in the past decade in the proportions of expectant and new mothers who are dependent on income support has created a large client group with specific health and social support needs (Blackburn and Graham, 1995). In a needs-led service, research to identify the health needs of this and other community health practitioner user groups is of paramount importance. This chapter will report on a large survey of the health and lifestyles of mothers on income support with new babies. Its aims are twofold. First, it seeks to highlight the value of large-scale health and lifestyles studies to health visitors and other community health practitioners in their search for health needs and their struggle to provide responsive services for disadvantaged households. Second, it aims to offer practitioners an opportunity to update and extend their knowledge of the health and living standards of mothers in receipt of income support and the context within which they make and carry out their decisions about infant feeding.

The chapter will begin by looking at the contribution of large-scale health and lifestyle studies. It will then move on to introduce the *Achieving Lifestyle Change* study (Blackburn and Graham, 1995), a large-scale study of mothers on income support. It will discuss the backdrop to the study, highlighting an increase in the number of mothers on income support giving birth to babies, and their marked social and material disadvantage. Moving on, the chapter examines the study, describing the research design and some of the issues that arise in researching the health and lifestyles of mothers living in disadvantaged circumstances. It illustrates the interconnections between health, lifestyles and living standards in the lives of mothers on income support, through an examination of mothers' social and economic circumstances and infant feeding patterns. Last, it will discuss some of the implications for practice, highlighting how health visitors and other community practitioners can promote breastfeeding among mothers on income support.

The contribution of large-scale health and lifestyle studies

The 1990s have seen a proliferation of policies that place requirements on health care organisations and workers to search for and identify local health needs. Although these policies place no legislative requirements on health visitors, it is widely acknowledged within health visiting, and increasingly outside it, by employers, local health authorities and other local purchasers, that they are a key resource in the search for the health needs of local populations and user groups within populations. The universal accessibility of health visitors to the whole population of a GP practice list facilitates the search for health needs at a local level. Large-scale health and lifestyle studies can be a valuable resource for practitioners. A major contribution of large-scale studies, based on nationally representative samples, is that they provide a canvas on which to paint health patterns and trends. The statistics generated offer a national perspective on local data and can then be used by community practitioners to assess how well or how badly placed local people are in terms of their health and social circumstances compared with the nation as a whole. While local health profiling activities provide a unique opportunity to fine-tune the search for health needs, it is important to recognise that the framework for local health need assessments can be guided by large-scale studies that pinpoint key aspects and dimensions of health. Large-scale studies can offer health needs searches some direction from which to begin.

Large-scale health studies also act as a medium for establishing explanations concerning how different parts of the broad health picture fit together: how health status and health experience are connected to health behaviour and living standards. While, in the past, living standards and health behaviour were researched separately (Graham, 1996), more recent studies have attempted to reveal the ways in which living standards and other dimensions of inequality, including race, gender and disability, fit together to shape people's health behaviour and health experience (see for example, Blaxter, 1990; Graham, 1992). These studies point to the need for local health searching to encompass and tie together local data on health experiences, health behaviour and the social and material circumstances of people's lives.

The *Achieving Lifestyle Change* study is an example of a large-scale health and lifestyle study that can inform the practice of health visitors and other community practitioners. This study focused on a group of women and their households neglected in other health surveys – mothers on income support. Although mothers on income support with young babies represent a significant health service user group, little is known about their health and health behaviour. National health surveys frequently use social class as the focus for examining differences between social groups. As a growing number of people on benefits have never had a full-time job, a significant proportion of people are absent from health statistics because they cannot be allocated a social class using the conventional criteria of social class allocation based on current or last full-time occupation. Benefits status has rarely been a focus for enquiry in national health and lifestyle surveys, and claimant households typically make up too small a subgroup in local surveys to permit their health and lifestyle to be analysed separately from those of the rest of the local population. Yet their circumstances and experiences frequently differ from those of other households. The study provided an opportunity to document and explore the interconnections between the health, lifestyles and living standards of this disadvantaged group, using a nationally representative sample. In a needs-led service, research to identify the health needs of user groups such as mothers and their households on income support is of paramount importance.

Mothers on income support

Searching for and seeking to provide services that are responsive to the needs of low-income mothers has become increasingly important for several reasons. First, there has been a significant increase in the proportion of mothers and their families who are dependent on income support, the key safety net social security benefit. Between April 1996 and March 1997, an estimated 217 000 babies were born to mothers in receipt of income support (DSS, 1997a). The proportion of babies born to mothers on income support has increased sharply over the past decade: in 1988, a fifth of babies were born to mothers in receipt of income support (DSS, 1989); by 1997, this figure had increased to about a third (DSS, 1997a). The number of households with children in receipt of income support has also risen. Between 1979 and 1996, there has been a three-fold increase in the number of households with children in receipt of income support, from 0.5 million to 1.5 million (DSS, 1980, 1997a).

These figures hide the diversity that exists within mothers' financial situations. Some groups of mothers are more likely than others to find themselves dependent on social security benefits such as income support. These include black and ethnic minority mothers, lone mothers and mothers who are themselves disabled or who are caring for a disabled adult or child in the household. High rates of unemployment among black and minority ethnic households leave them at high risk of financial poverty. The evidence suggests that while over half of Pakistani/Bangladeshi/Indian households and over a third of black African and black Caribbean households are dependent on income support, the comparable figure for white households is less than a fifth (DSS, 1997a, b). Like ethnic grouping, family structure also shapes people's dependence on benefits. In 1994–95, 64 per cent of all lone-parent families with dependent children (of which 9 out of 10 are lone mothers) were in receipt of income support compared with 10 per cent of two-parent families with dependent children (DSS, 1997a). Disability also increases the risk of low income and dependence on social security benefits. The Office of Populations, Censuses and Surveys' disability survey (Martin and White, 1988) found that a third of families with a disabled adult, compared with a quarter of families without a disabled adult, had a low income, that is, an income less than half the average income.

An increase in the proportion of mothers and their households in receipt of income support has been accompanied by a deterioration in their financial circumstances. While real incomes for the population as a whole have increased, some groups have not benefited from real rises in income. Since benefits have been linked to prices instead of wages, the income of those dependent on benefits has fallen behind that of the working population (Hill, 1995). On average, the income of income support claimants fell, in real terms, by 11 per cent between 1987 and 1991, and the poorest 10 per cent of households are now worse off than they were a quarter of century ago (Goodman and Webb, 1994).

A number of studies suggest that income support scale rates are inadequate to cover the basic needs of households with children. Oldfield and Yu (1993), after estimating the minimum costs of a child in the 1990s, compared these estimated costs against benefit scales. They concluded that rates of income support – the social security safety net – are set too low and would need to be 30 per cent higher if they were to provide a basic standard of living for parents and children. Further evidence on the inadequacy of benefits is available from a study of the diets and nutritional needs of expectant and new mothers (Dallison and Lobstein, 1995). This study indicated that a large proportion of low-income mothers regularly missed meals and a third ate diets that fell below 'seriously deficient' levels for five or more of the 10 vitamins and minerals measured in the study. On average, low-income new mothers were spending half the amount per week per person (£10.09) on food that was recorded as the national average weekly spending (£21.01).

Studying new mothers on income support

Against this background of increasing poverty among mothers dependent on income support, the *Achieving Lifestyle Change* study set out to fill a gap in existing knowledge about the health and health behaviour of this health service user group. In addition to providing participants with an opportunity to describe their health and living standards, the survey also offered a window through which some health behaviours could be examined. The survey focused on two health behaviours regarded as being important determinants of child and adult health: infant feeding and cigarette smoking. Within the confines of this chapter, only the data on infant feeding will be discussed, the findings on cigarette smoking being reported elsewhere (Blackburn and Graham 1995; Graham and Blackburn, 1998).

The survey was conducted with the support of three community Trusts in three Midlands cities. The sampling frame for the study consisted of new mothers in receipt of income support who lived within the boundaries of the three Trusts and who had delivered singleton babies during an 8-month period in 1994. As mothers would be asked to describe and comment on their experiences of early motherhood, the sampling criteria required that mothers should be living with their babies at the time of filling in the questionnaire (thus excluding mothers with babies in special care baby units or who were not living with their babies for child protection reasons). Mothers were asked to participate in the study by their family health visitor, who explained the study to them and gained their consent.

The health visitors' involvement was central to ensuring the success of the study for a number of reasons. First, health visitor contact with families at the birth visit provided an opportunity to access and recruit a sample of mothers that was large enough to allow a meaningful statistical analysis of the data. Second, health visitors provided the key to obtaining the mothers' co-operation and consent. As health workers familiar to and trusted by most families, they could contribute to increased questionnaire completion and return rates by explaining the importance of the study to the mothers.

Involving health visitors in the recruitment process required permission from the Trusts and clearance from local ethics committees. In addition, it demanded an extensive health visitor training programme, designed to brief over 300 health visitors across three NHS Trusts about the study and about recruitment methods. Like many research studies, this study was dependent on how those who act as intermediaries between potential research participants and researchers – in this case health visitors – evaluate the proposed study and assess its usefulness in terms of their work. Negotiating access to research participants is often multilayered. While local ethics committees and Trust managers form the first links in the chain between researchers and potential research participants, it is often those further down the chain, for example health visitors, who hold the key to successful sample recruitment.

Health visitors recruited mothers at the birth visit. Where this was not possible, an invitation was issued at the next visit. To facilitate the participation of mothers whose first language was not English, contracts were set up with interpreting agencies to provide information in the main languages spoken by the mothers in the three localities and to provide linkworkers/interpreters to assist mothers who wished to take part in the study. Mothers who wished to participate were invited to complete a postal questionnaire or to complete a questionnaire with an interviewer or linkworker/interpreter. This latter option provided an opportunity for a group of women who are frequently excluded from surveys to take part. By failing to encompass this group of women, many surveys are likely to under-estimate social and material disadvantage and poor health experiences in the group. By including this group, the study sought to incorporate women who, because of poor access to jobs and the labour market, have the poorest social and economic circumstances.

Of the 1016 mothers who met the criteria for inclusion, 152 mothers (15 per cent) agreed to participate but did not complete a questionnaire or interview, and 81 mothers (8 per cent) refused to participate; 783 (77 per cent) completed a questionnaire or interview. This high response rate reflects the commitment of the participating health visitors and compares favourably with the rates achieved by other surveys of disadvantaged groups. A check on the characteristics of non-responders suggested that there were no significant differences between non-responders and the mothers who took part.

The majority of participants (93 per cent) self-completed a postal questionnaire, with a small proportion completing a questionnaire with an interviewer in English (4 per cent) or with a linkworker or interpreter in their own language (3 per cent). In recognition of the mothers' contribution, anyone who completed a questionnaire, alone or with assistance, received a £10 voucher to thank them for their help, as well as a newsletter summarising the project findings. For the majority of mothers, questionnaires or interviews were completed by the time their babies were 8 weeks old. Questionnaires collected detailed information on infant feeding practices and smoking behaviours, as well as material circumstances, caring responsibilities, health, lifestyle and social support networks. Where possible, standardised and validated measures were used.

Before moving on to examine patterns of infant feeding, it is useful to look briefly at the mothers' social and economic circumstances. Not only do these form the back-drop to and provide a way of understanding the context within which mothers on low incomes feed and care for their babies, but they also remind us that they do so in conditions of hardship.

The mothers' circumstances

The majority of mothers (83 per cent) identified themselves as white (white UK, white other or Irish). Of the remaining mothers, 10 per cent described themselves as black (black African, black Caribbean or black other), 4 per cent as South Asian (Indian, Pakistani, Bangladeshi or Vietnamese) and 4 per cent as being of mixed parentage or of another ethnic group. Just over half of the mothers (53 per cent) were under the age of 25, and over two-thirds (69 per cent) were caring for at least one other child in addition to their new baby.

The mothers' demographic characteristics suggest a group marked by personal disadvantage. A third of mothers (34 per cent) had never had a full-time occupation. Among lone mothers, this increased to 50 per cent. Among mothers living in a cohabiting relationship (with a partner/ husband), almost a third (29 per cent) had partners who had never had a full-time job. As allocation to a social class is based on the current or last full-time occupation of the head of household, this meant that a third of the mothers could not be allocated to a social class group. This high- lights how health and social statistics based on social class measures are unlikely to reflect the social and health expe- riences of a growing number of people who have never been in full-time employment. This suggests that practitioners using these sets of statistics as a means of understanding health patterns should be aware of their limitations.

Data on the mothers' living standards reveal a group with poor access to important material health resources. Measures of housing tenure indicate that mothers were heavily clustered in the rented sector, with fewer than 1 in 5 (17 per cent) living in owner-occupied accommodation. The extent of the mothers' housing disadvantage becomes clear when these data are compared with national data suggesting that 7 out of 10 households with children (69 per cent) live in owner-occupied accommodation (Office for National Statistics, 1997). Among mothers in the survey, only 41 per cent had access to a car or van; nationally, the corresponding figure is 7 out of 10 (Office for National

Statistics, 1997). There were significant differences in housing and car/van ownership between Asian and other mothers in the sample. Among Asian mothers, those in the rented sector were in the minority (45 per cent). Of other mothers, the proportion living in the rented sector was twice as high (Office for National Statistics, 1997). Access to a car was also affected by ethnicity and household structure. Asian mothers living with a partner or with their parents were most likely to have access to a car/van (69 per cent) and black mothers on their own or with a partner least likely (28 per cent).

Just over half (51 per cent) of the mothers had been in receipt of income support for more than 2 years, a fifth (21 per cent) having been dependent on income support for more than 5 years. Research suggests that families experience a sharp deterioration in living standards when they have been on benefits for more than 1 year (Heady and Smith, 1989). Consumer durables such as washing machines wear out, and clothes and shoes need renewing but are difficult to replace on current benefit rates. Mothers' assessments of their financial well-being captures some of the stresses associated with caring for children on income support. Nine out of 10 mothers (92 per cent) reported that they had money worries, about half the mothers (58 per cent) worrying quite often or all the time about money. Money worries were related to the length of time that mothers had been on income support, these increasing as the length of time on income support rose.

Mothers' experiences were characterised by poor health. National surveys of self-assessed health suggest that most women assess their own health as being good (Joint Health Surveys Unit, 1997). Mothers in the survey, however, reported significantly lower rates of good health in pregnancy and the postnatal period. There were no ethnic group differences in self-assessed health. One in 10 mothers (11 per cent) described a longstanding disability or illness. For many women, poor psychosocial health was a daily feature of their lives. Three-quarters (73 per cent) of the mothers were experiencing some degree of depression at the time of data collection. A substantial proportion also reported that they had felt depressed during their pregnancy. Some mothers were also caring without adequate social support, around a third of the mothers in a cohabiting relationship lacking access to a supportive relationship with a partner.

Taken together, these measures of health and social circumstances indicate a group of mothers caring for and making decisions about their own and their children's health in very disadvantaged circumstances. Against this background, the following sections look at the mothers' infant feeding decisions and behaviour.

Infant feeding

An important feature of the study was to fill in gaps in the knowledge about the health behaviour of women on income support by mapping the infant feeding patterns. Infant feeding practices are regarded as important determinants of child and adult health. Breastfeeding is generally promoted as the preferred method of infant feeding and is thought to provide the best source of nutrition for newborn infants, increasing resistance against gastrointestinal infections in the early months of life and reducing the incidence of allergies (DoH, 1994). The infant feeding patterns evident in the 1990 *Infant Feeding* survey (White *et al.*, 1992) suggest low rates of breastfeeding among mothers in low social classes. However, as highlighted earlier, social class data can obscure patterns among low-income groups by excluding a significant proportion of people from the statistics. The study provided a unique opportunity to map infant feeding patterns among mothers dependent on income support. This section describes some of the main findings most relevant to health visitors, looking first at sources of advice and influence in pregnancy and mothers' beliefs on infant feeding and feeding intentions in pregnancy, and second, at the incidence and duration of breastfeeding.

Kinship and friendship networks appeared to exert an important influence on infant feeding patterns. Among mothers participating in the survey, the majority were caring for their babies within social networks in which bottle feeding rather than breastfeeding was the norm. Fewer than 1 in 10 mothers (8 per cent) reported that they were living in social networks in which breastfeeding was the norm. A small proportion – just over a third (38 per cent) – said that they had been breastfed themselves as babies. Mothers were asked about the sources of advice and information on infant feeding to which they had access in pregnancy. A substantial minority reported that they did not recall receiving any advice on infant feeding from professional or lay sources in pregnancy, a third (32 per cent) describing how they had not received any professional advice or information and a similar proportion (38 per cent) reporting that they did not receive any advice or information from lay sources. While it is likely that some of these mothers may have received advice but could not recall it, a failure to recall advice or information may suggest that mothers were not receiving repeated positive reinforcement of information or that the strategies used to give information were ineffective.

Looking more closely at the mothers' sources of information suggests, as one might expect, that midwives and health visitors were commonly reported sources of information. Two-thirds (66 per cent) of mothers recalled receiving information from a community midwife, just over half remembering receiving information from a hospital midwife (58 per cent) or a health visitor (54 per cent). The majority of mothers who recalled receiving professional advice rated that advice as helpful. Among lay sources of advice, their own mothers were the only source identified by the majority of respondents (57 per cent), although quite a large proportion recalled receiving advice and information on infant feeding from a friend (48 per cent) or partner (46 per cent). Black and Asian mothers were more likely than other mothers to describe receiving advice from sisters and that this source of advice was helpful.

Given that breastfeeding was not the norm among family and friends, what is striking is the mothers' positive attitudes to breastfeeding. Just over half of the mothers (53 per cent) regarded breastfeeding as the best method of infant feeding, fewer than 10 per cent viewing bottle feeding as best (breast/bottle equally good: 30 per cent; not sure: 9 per cent). However, breastfeeding was the intended feeding method of only 4 out of 10 mothers (40 per cent) (this figure including those who intended to give both breast and bottle feeds). Some ethnic differences were evident. Black mothers and mothers classified as mixed parentage/other ethnic group were more likely than Asian or white mothers to report that, during pregnancy, they had decided to breastfeed.

The incidence of breastfeeding is measured nationally by the proportion of babies who are put to the breast initially, even if they are put to the breast only once. In Great Britain, the incidence of breastfeeding is 63 per cent (White *et al.*, 1992). Among mothers on income support in this study, the corresponding figure was 44 per cent (Figure 7.1). Although lower than the national incidence of breastfeeding, this figure compares favourably with the breastfeeding incidence recorded among mothers in social class V (41 per cent).

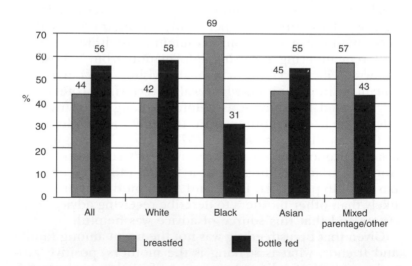

Figure 7.1   Incidence of breastfeeding (those who breastfed initially) by ethnic group

The proportion of mothers who put their babies to the breast initially was higher than the proportion who reported that, during pregnancy, they had intended to breastfeed. There were some significant ethnic group differences in the incidence of breastfeeding, black mothers having the highest incidence and white mothers the lowest (Figure 7.1). The incidence of breastfeeding was slightly higher among mothers of first babies than among mothers of second or subsequent babies, but these differences were not statistically significant and were less than those found nationally.

The proportion of all mothers who were breastfeeding when their babies were 6 weeks old was 22 per cent (Figure 7.2). This indicates that half (51 per cent) of the mothers who breastfed initially were still breastfeeding when their babies were 6 weeks old.

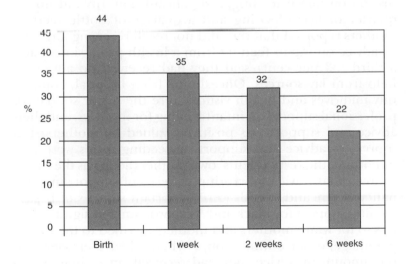

Figure 7.2   Percentage of mothers breastfeeding from birth to 6 weeks postpartum

Again, this compared favourably with breastfeeding duration patterns recorded in the *Infant Feeding* survey. Of those
mothers who initially breastfed but then gave up, giving
up breastfeeding was rarely a positive choice. Eight out of
10 of these mothers (84 per cent) reported that they would
have liked to have breastfed for longer. The main reasons
cited for switching to bottle feeding were similar to those
identified in the *Infant Feeding* survey: insufficient milk,
the baby would not suck, painful breasts or nipples and
maternal tiredness. Problems relating to breastfeeding were
also experienced by mothers who were able to overcome
these problems and continue breastfeeding. Mothers identified personal support – from their own mothers, partners, friends and health professionals – and extra rest as
the main ways in which they overcame such problems.

Looking more closely at patterns of professional and lay
support since leaving hospital suggests that while the majority
of mothers reported that they had received advice and information on infant feeding, a significant minority did not. A
quarter of breastfeeding and a quarter of bottle feeding
mothers reported that they did not recall receiving any help
or advice on infant feeding from a health professional, and
a third (33 per cent) said they had received no advice or
help from lay sources. Once home from hospital, community midwives and health visitors were the major sources of
professional support on infant feeding for mothers, and their
advice and support was positively valued by mothers. Lay
sources of advice and support on feeding issues were also
important, the respondents' own mothers acting as the major
source of lay advice. Mirroring patterns of support in pregnancy, sisters and friends were important sources of breastfeeding support for black and Asian women, but significantly
less so for white mothers and mothers ascribed to the mixed
parentage/other ethnic group. When asked their views on
the amount of advice they had received since their baby's
birth, only two-thirds of mothers (65 per cent) thought that
they had received the right amount of advice. This suggests
that there may be considerable scope for midwives and
health visitors to provide additional support to nursing
mothers in the postnatal period.

Influences on infant feeding

Researchers have investigated the factors associated with the initial choice of feeding method and the factors associated with the duration of breastfeeding. A common finding emerging from these studies has been that factors associated with the initial choice of breastfeeding are also associated with breastfeeding duration. These include higher social class, the experience of further/higher education or training, greater maternal age and support from a partner (Wright and Walker, 1983; Jones *et al.*, 1986; White *et al.*, 1992). These factors are important as they may be presented to health professionals during professional training and education courses as factors predictive of infant feeding behaviour and may be used to target resources at those most likely to succeed. The survey attempted to test out whether these correlates of breastfeeding in the general population were also associated with promoting and maintaining breastfeeding among mothers on income support.

The study identified a more complex picture than many other studies. Only a small cluster of factors found to be associated with breastfeeding in other studies were linked to both starting to breastfeed and maintaining breastfeeding among mothers on income support. These included ethnic group, school leaving age, further education and training experience, mothers' and partners' views about infant feeding and infant feeding intentions and beliefs. Ethnicity appeared to be an important factor, black mothers and mothers ascribed to the mixed parentage/other group more likely to breastfeed initially and to sustain breastfeeding for longer than Asian or white mothers. Mothers who stayed on at school beyond the age of 16 years and who had taken further education or training demonstrated higher breastfeeding incidence rates and longer duration rates. Among women with partners, those whose partners felt that the mother should breastfeed were more likely to breastfeed initially and to continue to breastfeed until at least 6 weeks after the birth.

In common with other studies, the survey found that mothers' infant feeding attitudes, experiences and intentions appeared to be the major predictors of infant feeding behaviour (White *et al.*, 1992). Confirming the evidence from other studies, most mothers carried out decisions about infant feeding made in pregnancy. Three-quarters of those who said they had decided during their pregnancy to breastfeed went on to breastfeed their babies initially, and three-quarters of those who had decided to bottle feed went on to bottle feed their babies after the birth. However, the study also highlights how some mothers changed their mind. A quarter of those who said they had decided in pregnancy to bottle feed put their babies to the breast initially, and a fifth of this group of mothers went on to breastfeed for 6 weeks or more. This suggests that while infant feeding decisions made in pregnancy are important, they may not, for some women, be fixed, some intending bottle feeders starting and maintaining breastfeeding once their baby is born.

Among mothers having a second or subsequent child, previous infant feeding experiences were important predictors of current infant feeding behaviour. Those mothers who had breastfed their oldest child until he or she was at least 6 weeks old were more likely initially to breastfeed their current baby and to continue to breastfeed until the baby was at least 6 weeks old. Again, the study highlighted that while previous infant feeding experiences are important, they do not determine current infant feeding choices for all mothers. Almost a third of those who had bottle fed their oldest child, initially breastfed their latest baby. A third of these mothers went on to breastfeed until their babies were at least 6 weeks old.

A range of factors were associated with initial breast-feeding but not with the duration of breastfeeding. Mothers most likely to feed initially were those aged 21 years or more. Although younger mothers were less likely to start breastfeeding, there was, in contrast with other research, no evidence to suggest that once they had started to breastfeed, they were less likely than other mothers to give up breastfeeding before their babies were 6 weeks old. Having a partner in whom the mother could confide was a further factor associated with starting breastfeeding. Once again, however, as this factor was not linked to maintaining breastfeeding, it cannot be assumed that mothers without confiding partners were any less likely to continue to breastfeed once they had started. The only independently predictive factor linked to maintaining breastfeeding, but not to breastfeeding initially, was living in owner-occupied rather than rented accommodation. Other living standard factors, or family structure, did not appear to be linked to infant feeding.

Conclusion and implications for practice

The study described in this chapter provided a unique opportunity to explore the health and reported health behaviour of a health visiting user group who have in the past been largely neglected by health researchers. This chapter discusses the health and lifestyles of mothers on income support. In doing so, it draws attention to the role of large-scale studies of health and lifestyle in helping practitioners to understand the health needs of user groups. These studies provide some direction for searching for health needs at the local level, pointing out important aspects and dimensions of health experiences and health behaviour. In addition, they can illustrate that health behaviours amount to more than simple choices about behaviour: they are rooted within material and social circumstances and social support networks. This suggests that local health needs searching must have mechanisms to allow health needs associated with living standards and lifestyles to be readily identified. Furthermore, large-scale health and lifestyle studies can generate comparative data against which the health of local people can be measured.

The study described here fills a gap in our information and knowledge about the health, lifestyles and living standards of mothers dependent on income support. It points out that mothers and their families living on income support have poor living conditions and poor physical and psychosocial health. Comparing these data with those from other surveys highlights that these mothers are considerably more disadvantaged materially, socially and in health terms than better-off groups. This material, social and health disadvantage was the context within which mothers on income support cared for and fed their babies. The evidence generated by the study contradicts a commonly held stereotype that this group of mothers are unlikely to breastfeed their babies: it pointed out that a substantial minority of mothers on income support did breastfeed. Just under half of mothers breastfed initially, and half of these mothers went on to sustain breastfeeding for 6 weeks or more. Importantly, this study suggests that predicting which mothers will start and sustain breastfeeding is likely to be difficult. Some of the factors identified in other studies as predictive of the initial choice and duration of feeding were not linked in the same way to breastfeeding behaviour among mothers on income support.

A more sensible and productive strategy for community health practitioners would be to regard all low-income mothers in pregnancy as potential breastfeeders rather than potential bottle feeders. Improving local and national breastfeeding targets is likely to depend, at least in part, on bringing about gains in breastfeeding among low-income women. Nationally, even small improvements in breastfeeding rates among mothers on income support would raise the incidence of breastfeeding among this group so that it became a majority, rather than a minority, habit.

A key starting point may be to ensure that all mothers receive information and advice about breastfeeding during pregnancy and the postnatal period, in a form that they find helpful. A significant minority of mothers on income support may not receive, or may not recall receiving, any information or advice about infant feeding, including breastfeeding, from professional or lay sources. Finding ways of giving infant feeding information and advice, in ways that mothers find helpful and recall, is likely to be central to improving breastfeeding rates. The study highlights that finding sensitive ways of providing information on breastfeeding to all women during pregnancy – and not just to women who state an intention to breastfeed –

is likely to be important, if somewhat challenging. A significant number of mothers who state an intention to bottle feed change their minds on the birth of their babies. Moreover, some mothers who have bottle fed previous babies go on to breastfeed their latest babies. These mothers need professional and lay information and support in pregnancy.

As kinship and friendship networks appear to play a central role in providing support for women, particularly black women, with regard to infant feeding, finding ways of utilising them may be an important health promotion strategy. Few of the mothers in this study lived in social networks in which breastfeeding was the norm. Changing the 'norm' is likely to be slow and occur over a period of time as breastfeeding rates are slowly increased. In the meantime, finding ways of putting potential and actual breastfeeders in touch with local peers who are breastfeeding, or who have previously breastfed, may be a useful strategy. Using local women as breastfeeding peer counsellors has been shown to be an effective way of supporting breastfeeding women in local populations (Riordan, 1995).

Given that the study highlighted the personal disadvantage of the women, in terms of education and training, it is likely that broader strategies to promote breastfeeding will be required. This includes strategies and policies to enable young women to stay at school longer, receive further education and training, and enter the labour market in well-paid and secure employment. While health visitors and other community practitioners can have little direct influence on national policies to reduce women's personal disadvantage, they have a role to play locally, supporting initiatives that seek to improve women's educational opportunities (for example, schemes aimed at improving literacy and numeracy skills), and through their professional organisations, to make clear the links between personal disadvantage and infant feeding behaviour.

The study also pointed to the difficult material and social circumstances within which mothers feed and care for their babies. Although the provisional analysis of data reported here did not point to any associations between material circumstances and infant feeding behaviour, these conditions were linked to the mothers' smoking behaviour (Graham and Blackburn, 1998) and have been linked in other studies to poor health and unhealthy behaviour (for a comprehensive review of these studies see Blackburn, 1991; Benzeval *et al.*, 1995). These studies suggest that finding ways of helping mothers on income support and their households to maximise their income and access other important resources for health, such as childcare resources, safe play areas and social support networks, continues to be central to supporting low-income households and improving the general health and well-being of women and their families.

The study discussed here highlights that health visitors and other community health practitioners play an important role in research by acting as intermediaries between research participants and those who carry out research. In this study, health visitors facilitated the recruitment of a sample of mothers who are often excluded from research studies. For the health visitors involved, it meant taking on another commitment in addition to numerous other commitments and responsibilities. Hopefully, the discussion of this project shows that while health visitors and community practitioners not only have a duty to protect service users from unethical and exploitative research, they also play an important part in promoting research that generates information to inform the development of effective support services.

KEY POINTS

- Large-scale health and lifestyle surveys are a useful resource for those concerned with searching for health needs at a local level: they provide some direction to local data, offer comparative data and highlight the need to link health and living standards information together.

- Mothers on income support, a large user group of health services, care for and feed their babies in very disadvantaged circumstances.

- A substantial minority of mothers breastfeed their babies. This data counteracts a commonly held stereotype that they are very unlikely to breastfeed.

KEY POINTS (cont'd)

■ It is likely to be difficult to predict which mothers on income support will breastfeed. Sensible strategies for promoting breastfeeding among this group are likely to include ensuring that all mothers receive and can recall information in pregnancy about breastfeeding, using family and kin support networks to promote breastfeeding and campaigning for policies that improve women's personal disadvantage.

References

Benzeval M., Judge K. and Whitehead M. (1995) *Tackling Inequalities in Health: An Agenda for Action.* London: King's Fund.

Blackburn C. (1991) *Poverty and Health: Working with Families.* Milton Keynes: Open University Press.

Blackburn C. and Graham H. (1995) *Achieving Lifestyle Change: A Survey of Mothers on Income Support in Three Community NHS Trusts in the Midlands.* Coventry: Department of Applied Social Studies, University of Warwick.

Blaxter M. (1990) *Health and Lifestyles.* London: Routledge.

Dallison J. and Lobstein T. (1995) *Poor Expectations: Poverty and Undernourishment in Pregnancy.* London: NCH Action for Children/Maternity Alliance.

Department of Health (DoH) (1994) *Weaning and the Weaning Diet.* London: HMSO.

Department of Social Security (DSS) (1980) *Social Security Statistics.* London: HMSO.

Department of Social Security (DSS) (1989) *Social Security Statistics.* London: HMSO.

Department of Social Security (DSS) (1997a) *Social Security Statistics, 1997.* London: Stationery Office.

Department of Social Security (DSS) (1997b) *Family Resources Survey, Great Britain 1994–95.* London: Stationery Office.

Goodman A. and Webb S. (1994) *For Richer, for Poorer: The Changing Distribution of Income and Wealth in the United Kingdom, 1961–91.* London: Institute for Fiscal Studies.

Graham H. (1992) *Smoking Among Working Class Mothers with Children: Final Report.* Coventry: University of Warwick.

Graham H. (1996) Researching women's health work: a study of the lifestyles of mothers on income support. In Bywaters P. and McLeod E. (eds) *Working for Equality in Health*. London: Routledge.

Graham H. and Blackburn C. (1998) The socio-economic patterning of health and smoking behaviour among mothers on income support. *Sociology of Health and Illness*, **20**(2): 215–40.

Heady P. and Smith M. (1989) *Living Standards During Unemployment*, Vol. 1. London: HMSO.

Hill J. (1995) *Joseph Rowntree Foundation Inquiry into Income and Wealth*, Vol. 2. York: Joseph Rowntree Foundation.

Joint Health Surveys Unit (1997) *Health Survey for England 1995*, Vol. 1: *Findings*. London: Stationery Office.

Jones D., West R. and Newcombe R. (1986) Maternal characteristics associated with the duration of breastfeeding. *Midwifery* **2**(4): 141–6.

Martin J. and White A. (1988) *The Financial Circumstances of Disabled Adults Living in Private Households*. OPCS Survey of Disability in Great Britain, Report No. 2. London: HMSO.

Office for National Statistics (1997) *Living in Britain: Results of the 1995 General Household Survey*. London: HMSO.

Oldfield N. and Yu A. (1993) *The Costs of a Child: Living Standards for the 1990s*. London: Child Poverty Action Group.

Riordan R. (1995) Breast-feeding peer councillor programme. *Midwifery Matters* **66**: 9.

White A., Freeth S. and O'Brien M. (1992) *Infant Feeding 1990*. London: HMSO.

Wright H. and Walker P. (1983) Prediction of duration breastfeeding in primiparas. *Journal of Epidemiology and Community Health* **37**: 89–94.

8

Identifying Outcomes in Health Visiting: The Challenge for Research

Amanda Kelsey

This text has brought together a number of separate pieces of research that are all related in some way to the idea enshrined in the concept of 'the search for health needs' (CETHV, 1977). As explained in Chapter 1, this principle remains important because of policy requirements to assess needs prior to planning or delivering services to meet them. However, despite continued legislative emphasis on this idea (DoH, 1989a, 1997), what counts as a 'need' is left unclear.

One much-cited definition that has captured the spirit of the NHS and Community Care Act 1990 suggests that 'need is the ability to benefit from health care' (Stevens and Gabbay, 1991: 20). There are a number of difficulties with this definition, particularly the questionable assumption that need relates more closely to the potential of service provision than to the experience of the person whose possible needs are under consideration. Earlier chapters in this text have shown that lay perceptions may differ quite markedly from the 'official' perspectives used by service planners. Indeed, even the use of the term 'need' might lead to offence, particularly if applied to the healthy populations who are the usual target group for health-promoting interventions by public health nurses such as health visitors or school nurses (Cowley *et al.*, 1996).

However, one advantage of defining need as the ability to benefit from care is that it provides a starting point for identifying health outcomes, especially if it is assumed that clinical interventions directed at individuals are the priority of the health service. Also, the definition shows that, from a service planning perspective, the two issues of 'health need' and 'health outcome' are inextricably linked.

In the light of this background, this final chapter will focus on three issues. First, it will outline the legislative imperatives and policy context that has created such a heavy emphasis on the identification of health outcomes. Second, it will explore some of the key difficulties that arise when trying to identify the outcomes of a public health service such as health visiting. These insights are equally relevant to other community nurses, especially those who work in teams, focus upon groups or populations rather than individuals, or target a well population. Finally, it will suggest some possible ways of identifying outcome measures that are acceptable to clients, practitioners and commissioners of services.

Legislative imperatives

The publication of two White Papers in 1989 (DoH, 1989a, 1989b) and subsequent legislation under the NHS and Community Care Act 1990 began a far-reaching process of reform within the health service. In particular, *Working for Patients* (DoH, 1989a) proposed the introduction of competition within this large public service by the use of an internal market. While the major focus of this paper was on the provision of hospital care, another important part of the reforms entailed the introduction of GP fund-holding. These reforms have been reported in detail elsewhere (for example Glennerster and Le Grand, 1994), and are not the main focus of this chapter since they will soon be of historical interest only.

In 1997, the general election brought a change of government and new proposals for a so-called 'third way' of running the NHS in England (DoH, 1997). The centralised command and control approach of the 1970s is rejected, as is the post-1989 model of the internal market. Instead, a more collaborative approach is advocated, which, it is hoped, will lessen inequities of provision. The planning and provision of health care will remain separate, and 'funding for all hospital and community services, prescribing and general practice infrastructure will be brought together' (DoH, 1997: 3). Thus several types of care will be considered together and choices made about the relative importance of each. Community prevention and care will compete for priority with the sophisticated technological procedures undertaken in hospital, for example.

The proposed structure is directed towards dismantling the internal market; because of the renewed emphasis on collaboration, groups of primary care workers in the same locality will be required to plan services together. The proposals emphasise the involvement of community nurses with GPs in assessing needs and planning provision for local people. There are four levels of involvement from which Primary Care Groups can choose. At minimum, they simply inform the health authority of preferences, while at the most advanced level, they take responsibility for the entire planning process, including the management of the budget and delivering some services, as primary care Trusts (DoH, 1997). Even at that level, they will be expected to work within the health improvement programmes set up by health authorities.

Subsequent modifications are possible as details of the legislation are finalised and as it proceeds through parliament, so it is not proposed to review these proposals in more detail here. However, given the continued distinction between those authorities responsible for planning services ('commissioners') and those which deliver them, some background about the reforms that first separated planning or commissioning and provision will help to explain why outcome measures became, and remain, such an important issue.

Policy in context

The changes introduced in 1990 were undoubtedly complex and reflect wider influences. Mohan (1996) describes them as taking place at three levels: macro, meso and micro. Macro-level explanations are based on the effect of a global economy; meso-level explanations place the reforms in a national and political context; and micro-level explanations consider the effects on the processes within the UK health service. These include the drive for effective health care and outcome measures that is the subject of this chapter.

Commentary on the reforms of the early 1990s often begins by making reference to the supranational economy (Ham, 1992; Loveridge,1992; Saltman and von Otter, 1992; Le Grand and Bartlett, 1993; Mohan, 1996). Many countries faced escalating health expenditure (OECD, 1992, 1995) caused by increased public demand, ageing populations and the increasing sophistication and expense of developments in medical technology (Ham, 1992; Saltman and von Otter, 1992).

In 1989, health care expenditure in Britain accounted for only 5.8 per cent of the gross domestic product (Scheiber and Pouillier, 1991) compared with 12 per cent in the USA, for example. So, it was not simply a matter of cost: the reforms were ideologically driven (Glennerster and Le Grand, 1994; Mohan, 1996). Complete privatisation of the NHS would have been electorally unpopular. The reforms were intended to introduce market-like mechanisms into the planning and delivery of health care. These mechanisms have been referred to as quasi-markets (Glennerster and Le Grand, 1994; Le Grand and Bartlett, 1994; Glennerster, 1997). Although the UK is now 'stepping back' from this approach, similar market-driven systems of health care remain common throughout the developed world (Saltman and von Otter, 1992).

The NHS appeared to be reasonably cost-effective, but the service should achieve the best possible health for its patients and clients within an appropriate level of funding (Maxwell, 1984). In order to establish effectiveness, it was necessary to be certain what services, including health visiting, should be able to deliver, and to be able to demonstrate this delivery to commissioners. The concept of efficiency includes a dimension of value for money, which was emphasised under the internal market.

If a service is to give good value for money, decision-makers (such as purchasers) need to be able to understand exactly what is being done and to establish whether an equivalent level of health gain can be achieved with less money or whether further investment will produce greatly improved levels of health. Under the market-driven system, it was assumed that quality would be enhanced through competition because purchasers would seek the most effective, as well as the most efficient, services. One way of doing this was to use outcome measures; thus, the drive to identify and define service quality through this mechanism began in earnest once the contracting process was fully established.

The new policy context

The proposals contained in *The New NHS* (DoH, 1997) are deliberately aimed at moving away from competition and market forces, but the need to identify outcome measures will be, if anything, even more important under the new proposals. Effectiveness and quality are stressed as much as efficiency in the proposed framework for assessing performance (NHSE, 1998). The six elements of this framework separate out some of the component parts of health outcomes, as shown in Table 8.1.

The importance attached to these dimensions is further demonstrated by the introduction of a new form of accountability known as 'clinical governance' that is designed to create parity between measures of quality and expenditure. This includes a new statutory duty to ensure quality and high standards, which is to be supported by a new, special health authority known as the National Institute for Clinical Excellence. This authority will be expected to give a strong lead on clinical and cost-effectiveness and

Table 8.1   Framework for measuring the performance of the NHS

Areas and categories covered	Example performance indicators
I. Health improvement	The overall health status of populations, reflecting social and environmental factors and individual behaviour, as well as care provided by the NHS and other agencies.
II. Fair access	Access to services, as shown by surgery rates, early detection of certain diseases, people registered with NHS dentists and so on.
III. Effective delivery of appropriate healthcare	Includes health promotion, disease prevention, primary care management and compliance with quality standards.
IV. Efficiency	Maximising use of resources.
V. Patient/carer experience of the NHS	Including accessibility, co-ordination and communication and waiting times.
VI. Health outcomes of NHS care	To include success in reducing risk, reducing levels of diseases, in optimising functioning, improving quality of life and reducing premature death.

Source: Adapted from NHSE, 1998

to help develop new evidence-based service frameworks that embody the best practice in any given service. The need to define and identify outcome measures can clearly only increase as these proposals are rolled out.

Defining outcome measures

Simply expressed, health outcomes are the impact on health that interventions can be shown to have made. There are a number of commonly used definitions of outcome measure. Donabedian considers that outcomes depend on a broad understanding of health and welfare. He writes (1988: 1745) that:

Outcome denotes the effects of care on the health status of patients and populations.

A similar but more detailed definition (Last, 1995: 119) suggests that:

all the possible results that may stem from exposure to a causal factor or from preventive or therapeutic interventions; all identified changes in health status arising as a consequence of the handling of a health problem.

Although these are two commonly used definitions, one Australian publication lists over 15 further definitions (Baum, 1994). The number of definitions suggests that the application of the theoretical concept of measuring outcomes may require a range of approaches in practice. There are, however, three key criteria that appear in most definitions:

1. There must be a change in health status.
2. The changes must be attributable to the activity being evaluated.
3. The change must be measurable.

Each of these criteria presents health visiting with some challenges. Explaining why these challenges are particularly difficult for health visitors involves a brief consideration of the purpose of their role. As explained in Chapter 1 of this volume, health visitors' own understanding of their role is defined by the principles of health visiting; these are (CETHV, 1977; Twinn and Cowley, 1992):

- the search for health needs;
- the stimulation of an awareness of health needs;
- the influence on policies affecting health;
- the facilitation of health-enhancing activities.

These principles emphasise the maintenance and improvement of health, with recovery from illness having less emphasis placed upon it, yet the development of outcome measures has its origin in the management of the costs and quality of care of ill health. This may explain why more has been written about outcome measures for nursing (for example Bond and Thomas, 1991; Maggs and Snoxall, 1992; Pearson, 1993) and those writing about outcome measures for community practice find that little is written and progress is slow (Barriball and Mackenzie, 1993; Campbell *et al.*, 1995; Kelsey, 1995).

Having outlined both the challenges presented by the potential need to develop outcome measures and the purpose of health visiting, it is possible to consider these two dimensions together. This may clarify some of the sources of difficulty in measuring outcomes in health visiting.

Changing health status

Health visitors aim to sustain and enhance health, as stated in *The Principles of Health Visiting* (Twinn and Cowley, 1992). Sustaining health does not usually involve a change in health status but instead the prevention of a negative change. The complex nature of family health and the holistic approach of health visiting practice means that it is often not possible to predict exactly 'what it is' that is being prevented, so simply counting the existence of absence of problems will not demonstrate the fine detail of prevention (Cowley, 1995). It thus becomes difficult to measure outcomes for an important part of the work of health visitors, since maintenance of the *status quo* is not a change unless it is possible to measure the forces that would have negatively affected health had the preventive activities not taken place.

Many authors have attributed negative effects on health to socioeconomic and environmental factors (for example DHSS, 1980; Jarman, 1983; Whitehead, 1988; Whitehead and Dahlgren, 1991). Health visitors can usually only have a limited effect on such factors, but it is nevertheless important to show the links between health needs and health outcome. Deprivation can be measured and used in the context of measuring outcomes. For example, the challenges to health in a deprived area are likely to be more far reaching, so the interventions needed are likely to need to be greater and more complex in order to maintain or improve health. The outcomes may take longer to achieve and may be less obvious than in more privileged communities.

Outcome measures for effectiveness and efficiency need to include a consideration of the overall environment as well as specifically health-related factors. If this is not done, work in more privileged areas may appear to show a greater health gain, the logical result of which would be to increase resources where they seem to be most effective and to disinvest in deprived areas. Thus inequities in health could be increased.

Not only is the environment important, but also, where changes are achieved, they may be difficult to measure or may not be sustainable. For example, helping families to improve their diet is a reasonable aim, but it may be very difficult to measure any impact on health. Similarly, if the family's income changes, it may not be possible to sustain the improvements in diet, yet the change in income may not be related to health at all. Where the purpose of health care is to diminish the impact of ill health, it may be easier to use outcome measures to assess the effectiveness of care.

The problem of attribution

The level of deprivation in a community is an important influence on health, but so is access to information about health. One of the primary functions of health visitors is the provision of relevant health related information to enable clients to identify health needs or health-enhancing activities. These interventions are educative, and although they are likely to lead to changes in knowledge, they may not necessarily affect behaviour. In this situation, the health visitor has intervened and may indeed have produced a change – but not a change in health status.

Furthermore, health visitors are not the only source of health information; others include health education campaigns, newspapers, television programmes, family members, friends and self-help groups. Some of these sources can be more authoritative than others. Once clients have enough information, they may choose to act on it or not. Even if clients choose the course of action suggested by the health visitor, it is difficult to be certain that it was because of his or her intervention that the particular choice was made.

Physicians determine whether an outcome occurs as a result of an intervention or by chance by using control groups within a randomised controlled trial. The effects of the intervention can be measured by comparing effects in both intervention and control groups, provided the research method is both valid and reliable. Such experiments have been carried out to identify the impact of specific strategies on knowledge and long-term behaviour, but most of this work has been carried out in countries where there is no universal health visiting or public health nursing service, such as Canada or the USA. A systematic review of health visitor home visiting found good evidence of effectiveness for a number of different health needs (Robinson *et al.*, 1999). However, there are difficulties with transferring results to the UK: many of the studies used sample sizes that are too small to be conclusive and concentrated only on specific, high-risk populations. Attribution remains problematic even within the context of the randomised controlled trial, because it is not possible to control the wide influence of friends, family, media and other professionals involved with the experimental group.

Control groups could be used to test and develop outcome measures further in this country, but it would be difficult to justify continuing to offer the usual, universal service to one part of the community while withholding it from another. Indeed, many people feel that it would be unethical to suggest this. The alternative would be to use a similar community in another country without a universal health visiting service, but national and cultural differences could invalidate the comparisons. Thus cross-sectional comparisons for measurement purposes are problematic but may be suitable for particular areas of practice where national and cultural issues are less important.

It is increasingly common to find health visitors working as part of primary care teams. Where teamwork is well developed, it may be difficult to separate the work of the health visitor from that of other members of the team, in which case it is impossible to identify any outcomes specifically for the work of the health visitor. If health visitors cannot show that they have specific, relevant expertise aside from their general responsibilities as team members, the necessity for a discrete role and training becomes questionable. This problem is common to the majority of health care workers. The difficulty arises from the large number of factors and professional groups who influence health and is referred to by Long (1993) as 'the crucial issue of attribution'.

The problem of measurement

Longitudinal measurements are useful but they are also not without their difficulties: they face the same problems with attribution as do any studies of the effectiveness of health visiting. As shown by Graham and Blackburn's large-scale survey, reported in Chapter 7, longitudinal studies are time consuming and certainly need to last longer than the 3-year cycle over which health authorities and Primary Care Groups must develop their health improvement programmes. However, such baseline measurements are also needed in order to be able to assess the effect on health that any intervention has; more health surveys are needed to trace the pathways following normal life events to provide this information.

Most health visiting interventions occur after a major health and life event such as the birth of a baby or perhaps a major bereavement. Although clients' health could be measured in a variety of ways on first contact with the health visitor, it seems likely that such measurements will reflect not a true underlying state of health but rather the impact of recent events. It may, on first meeting, be difficult to separate the effects of, for example, tiredness and loss of appetite after an interrupted night's sleep from those arising from a routinely poor diet. Further-more, after a major event such as the birth of a baby, health should slowly improve with or without interven-tion. While attributing this gradual and normal improve-ment to the work of the health visitor could be misleading, the risk of problems arising if sufficient support is not available may be high for some vulnerable groups. The difficulty of identifying 'objective measures' by which to prioritise these individuals is well demonstrated by Appleton (see Chapter 4).

Finally, many of the changes in health that could possibly arise as a result of the work of health visitors may not become obvious for many years, or not at all, since preventing ill health is part of the work. Supporting clients' efforts to resist or stop smoking are an obvious illustration of this point. It is impossible to know how many people have failed to develop smoking-related diseases as a result of educational interventions.

Making valid outcome measurements for health visiting practice is, therefore, difficult for many reasons. As these examples show, the three key difficulties of demonstrating change, attribution and accurate measurement are all closely interlinked. However, as governments seek to ensure that the best possible use is made of taxpayers' money, health care interventions that are not demonstrably effec-tive in improving health may be vulnerable to funding cuts. Perhaps more important is the potential harm that may arise from delivering services that are not effective. Indeed, while some may feel that withholding the usual universal services for experimental purposes is unjustified, others may suggest that it is unethical to offer services that are not demonstrably safe and effective. Thus it is impor-tant to establish effectiveness and identify possible ways of assessing the outcomes of health visiting services.

Effects on practice

In an increasingly cost-conscious health service, there is the possibility that practice that is demonstrably effective will be funded more generously than practice that cannot demonstrate any effectiveness. This may lead to the holistic practice of health visiting being fragmented into activities and tasks that can be evaluated.

If practice becomes outcome driven, health visitors may find themselves concentrating on work with clients who are most likely to adopt the behaviours suggested. This would make the service inequitable and might discriminate against clients who could benefit most from it.

In order for an outcome measure to be valid, it should reflect the skills and practice of the health visitor. If the work could have been done by another professional group, either the outcome could have been, or was, achieved by a number of others and represents a team outcome, or the outcome is not a measure of health visiting practice. This issue may not be particularly relevant to either clients or politicians, but it is significant for the future of health visiting as a profession. Focusing service priorities solely upon the endpoint of the intervention may obscure the amount of time and skill needed. Without time for the background work of, for example, gaining a client's trust and building self-esteem, some obvious outcome measures, such as improving the child immunisation rate, may be difficult to achieve.

In order to fit into the annual contracting cycle, there may be a temptation to choose outcome measures that appear very simple and easily achievable rather than devoting efforts to longer-term strategies to improve individual or community health. *The New NHS* proposals stress health improvement and sustainability by introducing contracts over a 3-year rolling programme (DoH, 1997), and there is the promise of a greater emphasis on long-term public health measures (DoH, 1998). However, the parallel emphasis upon clinical effectiveness and associated pressure to identify clear outcome measures could still distract practitioners from working towards more fundamental improvements in health.

Finally, health visitors work not only with individuals and families, but also with communities. Community health may be studied by epidemiologists, and their methods could be used to identify outcome measures for these different levels of activity. Developments in this area have been hampered because so much health visiting work has been purchased by GP fundholders for their own practice populations. Most general practice populations are both too small and too geographically dispersed for such studies of health-related issues. With the advent of Primary Care Groups, which will typically take responsibility for populations of around 100 000 based on 'natural communities' (DoH, 1997), services could once more be commissioned across a wider area. The development of community health outcome measures could be promoted if data collection methods were standardised across an area and groups of practices.

Possible solutions

A number of problems with the definition and use of outcome measures have been outlined above. One way of overcoming many of the difficulties may be by using aggregated data. This would avoid any problems with determining outcomes for individuals and families, such as the temptation to work with clients who are more likely to 'co-operate', thus introducing an inequity in provision. There are two approaches to such aggregated data: one a 'population approach' and the other an aggregation of individually negotiated outcomes.

A population approach

This is based on the compilation of an accurate and detailed community profile. The profile is then used as a baseline measurement, and changes in community health status are measured by repeating the profiling process. Although this seems feasible, it could be difficult to assemble a profile that is sensitive enough to small changes in health to provide useful information. It might, however, be used to inform the setting of commissioners' priorities. In most general practice settings, the practice population would be too small to reduce the impact of confounding variables, and working with several local practice populations would require the profiles to be comparable.

An advantage of this approach is that it does not require a large amount of data collection on a daily basis; work could be done at the health visitors' discretion within the timeframe needed by commissioners.

Aggregating individually negotiated outcomes

Many health visitors negotiate with their clients in order to establish joint aims in maintaining or improving the health of clients as individuals or families. These will commonly include issues of child health such as nutrition, growth and development, immunisation, sleep and behaviour. Other issues include aspects of maternal health such as family planning, nutrition and body weight, smoking, rest and recreation, work, benefits and family finances. Other aspects of family health may also be considered; families may prefer to call such matters 'health issues' as focusing on the idea of 'need' may suggest an abnormality.

Within each aspect of health, individuals may have different needs for help and support, or none at all. However, health visitors could use the individually negotiated aims as a basis for outcome measures by aggregating the data. For example, the number of households in which smoking is an issue could be determined, together with the number in which support is being given for mitigating the effects of smoking (for example by smoking away from children) or reducing or stopping smoking. The number of households with whom the health visitor has undertaken some work on smoking then becomes the measure. This avoids assessing how successful he or she has been by only counting the number of people who have stopped smoking, since health visitors could not and would not wish anyone to stop smoking at their request.

Other health visiting activity might need documenting differently. For example, almost all visits to the mothers of new babies will include a discussion of nutrition and various other issues. This is the core work. In this case, the mother and health visitor may want to determine some joint goals such as continuing to breastfeed until the next clinic visit (if this seems reasonable). Such outcomes may vary from client to client but would have the nutrition of the baby in common. The number of households in which nutrition was discussed, together with the number in which jointly agreed goals were achieved, could then be ascertained. Over time, it might be possible to develop a more sophisticated hierarchy; for example, maintaining a satisfactory *status quo* in the area of infant nutrition could be scored, as could making certain improvements such as correcting a faulty feed preparation method. The scores could then be used to assess clients' progress towards the negotiated goals. Negative scores could be used to show that things had deteriorated, but if they were, it is important also to consider that clients' health behaviour is not under the control of the health visitor and negative scores may only mean that the goal needs to be reconsidered.

Although this system has much to recommend it, there are at least three major problems. The first is the amount of data collection in which the health visitors would become involved, and the second the possibility that local or national priorities might not feature in individual negotiations. The third issue is that unless the data collection methods were standardised, which could reduce sensitivity to local issues, there would be no real basis for comparison between areas. Even individually negotiated outcomes are more likely to be achieved in areas where living is less stressful, and there is a risk that further resources would be given to the more successful areas at the expense of areas that may be more deprived, less successful and actually in need of greater resources. A considered use of these measures could, however, meet the need for outcome measures and allow clients to continue to have a strong voice in determining their own health priorities as well as using the skills of health visitors to particular advantage.

A framework for the statement of outcome measures

A useful and robust framework for the statement of outcome measures has been developed by Long (1995, 1996). It is both sufficiently broad to encompass the wide range of health visiting work and specific enough to be useful. The framework has been used to develop outcome measures for specific health visiting activities and has been found to have much to offer (Long and Kelsey, unpublished data).

The framework consists of the following elements:

- A clear statement of the health issue to be addressed.
- A method of testing the baseline level of the dimension of health concerned, that is, the 'test'.
- A statement of the baseline measurement.
- The anticipated outcome, determined in negotiation between the client and health visitor. This may include measurements such as the frequency of attendance, the number of cigarettes smoked or other more subjective measures. Timescales may be usefully included in some measures.
- A comprehensive outline of what the health visitor has agreed to offer the client, including the skills to be used. A similar outline may be made for the client. In some circumstances, it may be appropriate to share the outline with clients, but the health visitor may consider adding a long list of skills later.
- It may be useful to record the category of health issue and position in the hierarchy if one exists. An example of such a hierarchy might be: maternal health, mental health, isolation or child health, nutrition, breastfeeding, timing.

This framework is flexible enough to be able to include individual, family or community health issues, although the negotiations necessary to ensure adequate representation in and agreement with a community may be demanding. It can be used for small-scale interventions or for supporting more major health-related change. It is sensitive to the circumstances of individual practice and the choice of aims and type of support made by clients or health visitors. However, the effect of this flexibility is also to leave much of the work of determining the outcome up to the clients and health visitors. Establishing suitable baseline measures may be demanding, depending on what is to be evaluated. For example, an improvement in self-esteem would be a legitimate aim for clients and health visitors but would be difficult to measure, and a less complex issue from which self-esteem might be built could be chosen, for example taking more exercise, resuming an interest, learning something new or finishing some uncompleted task. Clients may have their own versions of these proxies for measuring improvements in self-esteem, which could be used.

During 1993 and 1994, the framework was tried by a group of experienced health visitors, and outcome measures were developed in areas such as nutrition and the management of minor childhood ailments. There were no clients involved in the group, which meant that the group focused on professionally determined issues, but it was possible to use the framework within a wide range of areas of practice, indicating that it could be useful at a practical level.

Possibilities for the future

The development of outcome measures for health visiting is still at an early stage. Although it may not be an essential part of the evaluation of practice, it is to be hoped that outcome measures, if they are needed, will serve the needs of clients, the profession and the purchaser reasonably equally.

The development of a comprehensive nursing thesaurus would enable the construction of hierarchies of health-related behaviours. An overall thesaurus of health-related terms, incorporating those developed specifically for nursing use, is now available in the UK (Cowley and Casey, 1995). However, it is not widely in use, and nursing terms have not been separately tagged since the aim was to promote multidisciplinary working through a single shared language in computerised information systems. An alternative thesaurus is being developed by the International Council of Nurses (Clark, personal communication, 1998), and this may provide the necessary basis for research.

A comprehensive thesaurus would allow the recording of anonymised aggregated data about outcomes negotiated or achieved with individual clients, so that the amount of health visiting activity within the area of, for example, mental health, family planning or perhaps nutrition could be demonstrated. Such a project would require substantial investments of time, money and expertise but would clarify health visiting work.

Perhaps the question that remains is whether such an investment in quality assurance as expressed by outcome measures would be better used to develop further services for clients. This question once again raises the problem of the tension between cost and quality of care that underlies much recent health care reform. This tension applies as much to health visiting as it does to other areas of health care, with the additional problems raised by the health-promoting nature of the work. Evaluation, of which outcome measures can form a part, can be neglected only at the peril of the service.

KEY POINTS

- An emphasis on measuring outcomes has arisen because of economic and competitive pressures highlighted by the internal market introduced into the NHS in the early 1990s. The identification of health need is a necessary preliminary base from which to develop outcome measures.

- Legislation to dismantle this market emphasises effectiveness and quality as much as efficiency. It introduces a new form of accountability known as 'clinical governance' and a framework of indicators for assessing performance; these again bring the measurement of outcome to the fore.

- Health visiting practice is preventive and holistically directed at well individuals, families and the wider community. This is considered to be necessary to respond to the needs of clients and to promote public health. Outcome measures are possible in situations that meet the three criteria of changed status, clear attribution and measurability. These are difficult to meet without fragmenting health visitors' everyday practice or denying clients' preferences.

KEY POINTS (cont'd)

- If practice becomes outcome driven, health visitors may find themselves concentrating on work with clients who are most likely to adopt the behaviours suggested. This would make the service inequitable and might discriminate against clients who could most benefit from it.

- Suggestions for progress in measuring outcomes include ways of aggregating data from the whole area or across the health visiting caseload; this takes account of health visitors' wider responsibilities for public health and allows clients' views to be incorporated.

Acknowledgement

I would like to acknowledge the help of Andrew Long of the Outcomes Clearing House at the Nuffield Institute for Health, and of the group of experienced health visitors who worked with us to try out the framework's suitability for use in health visiting.

References

Barriball L. and Mackenzie A. (1993) Measuring the impact of nursing interventions in the community: a selective review of the literature. *Journal of Advanced Nursing* **18**: 401–7.

Baum F. (1994) Introduction. In *Health Outcomes in Community Health.* Adelaide: South Australian Health Research Unit.

Bond S. and Thomas L.H. (1991) Issues in measuring outcomes of nursing. *Journal of Advanced Nursing* **16**: 1492–502.

Campbell F., Cowley S. and Buttigieg M. (1995) *Weights and Measures: Outcomes and Evaluation in Health Visiting.* London: HVA.

Council for the Education and Training of Health Visitors (CETHV) (1977) *An Investigation into the Principles of Health Visiting.* London: CETHV.

Cowley S. (1995) In health visiting, the routine visit is one that has passed. *Journal of Advanced Nursing* **22**(2): 276–84.

Cowley S. and Casey A. (1995) The language of community nursing. In Littlewood J. (ed.) *Advances in Community Nursing.* Edinburgh: Churchill Livingstone.

Cowley S., Bergen A., Young K. and Kavanagh A. (1996) Identifying a framework for research: the example of needs assessment. *Journal of Clinical Nursing* **5**(1): 53–62.

Department of Health (DoH) (1989a) *Working for Patients*. Cmnd 555. London: HMSO.

Department of Health (DoH) (1989b) *Caring for People*. Cmnd 849. London: HMSO.

Department of Health (DoH) (1997) *The New NHS: Modern, Dependable*. Cmnd 3809. London: Stationery Office.

Department of Health (DoH) (1998) *A First Class Service: Quality in the New NHS*. London: Stationery Office.

Department of Health and Social Security (DHSS) (1980) *Inequalities in Health: Report of a Research Working Group* (The Black Report). London: DHSS.

Donabedian A. (1988) The quality of care: how can it be assessed. *Journal of American Medical Association* **260**(12): 1743–8.

Glennerster H. (1997) *Paying for Welfare: Towards 2000*. Hemel Hempstead: Harvester Wheatsheaf.

Glennerster H. and Le Grand J. (1994) *The Development of Quasi-markets in Welfare Provision*. STICERD discussion paper No. WSP/102. London: LSE/STICERD.

Ham C (1992) *Health Policy in Britain* (3rd edn). Basingstoke: Macmillan.

Jarman B. (1983) Identification of underprivileged areas. *British Medical Journal* **286**: 1705–9.

Kelsey A. (1995) Outcome measures: problems and opportunities for public health nursing. *Journal of Nursing Management* **3**: 183–7.

Last J.M. (1995) *A Dictionary of Epidemiology* (3rd edn). Oxford: Oxford University Press.

Le Grand J. and Bartlett W. (1994) *Quasi-Markets and Social Policy*. Basingstoke: Macmillan.

Long A.F. (1993) *Issues in Outcome Measurement*. Outcomes Briefing, Introductory Issue. Leeds: Nuffield Institute for Health.

Long A.F. (1995) *Clarifying and Identifying the Desired Outcomes of an Intervention: The Case of Stroke*. Outcomes Briefing No. 5. Leeds: Nuffield Institute for Health.

Long A.F. (1996) *Exploring Outcomes within Audit*. Outcomes Briefing No. 7. Leeds: Nuffield Institute for Health.

Long A. and Kelsey A. (unpublished) Outcome Measures and Health Visiting. PhD thesis jointly funded by NE Thames LORS Fund and Yorkshire region R&D.

Loveridge R. (1992) The future of health care delivery – markets or hierarchies? In Loveridge R. and Starkey K. (eds) *Continuity and Crisis in the NHS*. Buckingham: Open University Press.

Maggs C. and Snoxall S. (1992) *A Critical Review of the Literature on Outcomes in Nursing Practice and Management: A Report to the Department of Health*. London: HMSO.

Maxwell R. (1984) Quality assessment in health. *British Medical Journal* **12**(5): 1470–2.

Mohan J. (1996) Accounts of the NHS reforms: macro-, meso- and micro-level perspectives. *Sociology of Health and Illness* **18**(5): 675–98.

NHS Executive (NHSE) (1998) *The New NHS: Modern and Dependable: A National Framework for Assessing Performance – Consultation Document*. London: NHS Executive.

Organisation for Economic Cooperation and Development (OECD) (1992) *The Reform of Health Care: A Comparative Analysis of Seven OECD Countries*. Health Policy Studies No.2. Paris: OECD.

Organisation for Economic Cooperation and Development (OECD) (1995) *Internal Markets in the Making: Health Systems in Canada, Iceland and the United Kingdom*. Health Policy Studies No. 6. Paris: OECD.

Pearson A., Hocking S., Mott S. and Riggs A. (1993) Quality of care in nursing homes: from the residents' perspective. *Journal of Advanced Nursing* **18**: 20–4.

Robinson J.J.A. (1998) The Effectiveness of Domiciliary Health Visiting: A Systematic Review of the Literature. Presentation at RCN Health Visitor Forum Conference. London, 30 May 1998.

Saltman R. and von Otter C. (1992) *Planned Markets and Public Competition*. Buckingham: Open University Press.

Schieber G. and Pouillier J.P. (1991) International health spending: issues and trends. *Health Affairs* **10**: 106–16.

Stevens A. and Gabbay J. (1991) Needs assessment needs assessment. *Health Trends* **23**(1): 20–3.

Twinn S. and Cowley S. (eds) (1992) *The Principles of Health Visiting: A Re-examination*. London: UKCC/HVA.

Whitehead M. (1988) *The Health Divide*. London: Penguin.

Whitehead M. and Dahlgren G. (1991) What can be done about inequalities in health? *Lancet* **338**: 1059–63.

Index

Page numbers printed in **bold** type refer to figures; those in *italic* to tables or boxed material (key points).